Preface

The Sleep Nanny® philosophy is that no two children are the same, therefore you need a plan to help your child sleep and that plan should be tailored to suit your child and your family. Most people choose the method they most like the sound of rather than the approach that will be most effective and suited to their child.

There are many great sleep books out there by experts with different philosophies. For example, Richard Ferber is famous for his style of controlled crying technique, often confused with Marc Weissbluth's extinction or cry-it-out method which is actually very different. Gina Ford offers a very harsh and regimented approach which can work for some but for most, it is too unrealistic because children are human, not robots. William Sears is all about attachment parenting including co-sleeping, baby wearing and everything being baby-led. Elizabeth Pantley claims to have a 'no-cry' solution but this is selling an impossible dream because all changes to a baby's routine will be met with some degree of crying. It is how they communicate and express frustration. There are many gentle methodologies in between by the likes of Kim West, Tracy Hogg, Jodi Mindell and others, all of whom have a book on the shelves.

Some parents get lucky and happen to choose the right book or method that suits their parenting style and, coincidently, it works with their child's temperament which is probably quite an easy-going one. Many parents however, read everything, try everything, listen to everyone else's success stories but still cannot find something that works for them. They feel like they have a 'tricky sleeper' and often give up hope and prepare for the long haul of sleepless nights because they think they cannot be helped.

I decided to write this book to give parents an alternative approach to sleep training their babies or young children. Rather than try, guess or half-heartedly attempt something you have read or heard, wouldn't it be so much more powerful to be able to actually work out what THE best way is for YOUR child and your family? To put yourself firmly in the driving seat and be able to take control of the situation without any doubts or second-guessing?

This book will

- Help you to identify your child's temperament and personality
- Teach you about the science of sleep in young children to give you an understanding as to why they do what they do
- Enable you to match up the most suitable sleep training approach with your child's personality and your parenting philosophy
- Explain the importance of consistency
- Show you how to implement a plan successfully
- Uncover the importance of your role in your child's sleep journey
- Empower you to take action and feel in control

I did not want to write a baby sleep book like most other specialists in my field write, telling parents how to do it in their style, their method or their variation or twist on an existing philosophy. The reason being is that it wouldn't matter which angle I came from, it would still only be suited to a small number of parent/child combinations. From that, the idea for 'The Sleep Nanny System' was born. I realised I could offer parents the information that they need to work out what is right for them.

Contents

Introduction – My Story   page 7

Is This Book For You?   page 11

Secure Attachment   page 13

The Science Behind Sleep – Circadian
rhythms, sleep cycles, partial arousals,
sleep is a learned skill   page 15

Newborn Sleep   page 19

Identifying Your Child's Temperament   page 25

Understanding Sleep Training Methods   page 29

Routine   page 41

Sleep Crutches   page 43

Early Risers   page 45

Naps – More on naps and their importance   page 49

Transitioning Naps   page 53

Ditching The Dummy   page 57

Night Weaning   page 63

Self Settling   page 69

Consistency   page 71

Contents continued...

Average Sleep Needs By Age   page 75

Sleep And Wakeful Windows   page 77

How To Keep Your Child In
Their Own Bed All Night   page 79

How To Get Yourself Back To Sleep
After A Disturbance   page 85

Sleep Regressions, Developmental
Leaps And Fussy Phases   page 89

Nightmares, Night Terrors or
Something Else?   page 93

Teething And Sleep   page 99

Siblings And Sleep   page 101

Parenting And Sleep   page 103

Implementation   page 105

Troubleshooting – The Baby Sleep Blueprint™   page 107

Travel Tips   page 109

Daylight Savings – Clock Changes   page 113

Imperfect Parenting   page 117

Your USP (Unique Sleep Plan™)   page 119

Introduction - My Story

I am Lucy Shrimpton and I live in the south of England with my husband and two children. When we had our first child we had no idea what to expect in terms of sleep. Things started off pretty well because our little boy got himself into a nice rhythm with his feeds and he began to take a long stretch of sleep in the night after just a few weeks. By around six weeks he didn't even need a night feed as he was quite large and must have had a good capacity to go longer at night. We thought we had it sussed or at least that we were very lucky. I recall someone saying 'ha ha, just wait, that won't last' to which I remained calm and slightly smug, thinking of course it will last, why wouldn't it? There can be all kinds of reasons why you can get off to a good start like this and then it seems to come unstuck further down the line. At the time, I blamed it on the fact that we had a house guest for around five weeks which must have disrupted our little boy somehow and affected his sleep, as well as a new reliance on a dummy during the day (which had only been for bedtime before). Maybe this did have some affect on him or maybe it was not relevant at all, but what I do know now is that it couldn't have been the sole cause of the sleep difficulties we went on to endure for around four months!

With a new baby due to arrive, we knew we had to take action so we found some professional help to address our eldest's sleep difficulties which mostly consisted of early rising and frequent night waking as well as refusing to nap. We were exhausted! We also took some newborn advice to help us get off to a good start and not go down the same path with number two.

Within just one night of our sleep plan, our little boy slept through the night and within a week we stretched out his early starts to 6 a.m. and then to 7 a.m. within two weeks. It was incredible. Naps continued to be a bit of a challenge for a month or so and there were times when I thought the nap process would just not work for us, but I stuck with it and we got there in the end.

What I had learned made so much sense and yet was not obvious, so no wonder I hadn't found the answers in the books I had read. In the meantime, we made lots of progress with the new baby and shaping her sleep habits for the long term. Having just overcome the difficulties with a toddler's sleep, I was right at the start again with a newborn and determined to do things a little differently this time. It made the world of difference.

The whole topic of infant sleep became a passion of mine as I was fascinated by what I had learned and experienced first hand. Every time I spoke with a parent who was suffering like we had, I just wanted so desperately to be able to help them and enable them to experience life on the other side because it can be so much better and done so quickly! Someone at my children's nursery told me about a mother of a two-year-old who had never slept through the night and how she always looked so exhausted. That was it. I couldn't contain myself any longer. I needed to help these people, so I began my journey to learn everything there is to know about young children and sleep and become a certified and licensed professional.

I trained with one of the world's leading experts in infant sleep and the most comprehensive training programme available in this field of expertise. After many months of study, examination and test cases, I felt ready to serve tired parents everywhere. I also completed a diploma in maternity and child sleep consulting and continue to study and maintain my up-to-date knowledge.

My experience as a professional and as a mother has taught me so much and will only continue to do so with every new family I meet and every challenge I face as a mother too. I never want to stop learning because there is always another perspective, another challenge, another solution.

I spent a week in hospital after a difficult delivery with our eldest. He was in the Neonatal Intensive Care Unit (NICU) for a few days and then in the Transitional Care Unit (TCU) with me. The sleep deprivation I experienced during that time was horrendous. It was initiated by hospital staff moving me in the middle of the night after I had just got to sleep for the first time in two days. Given the traumatic experience I had been through, this sleep was needed. It was the beginning of the most difficult week of my life! Apparently they use sleep deprivation as a form of torture in some countries and I now know why. It does crazy things to your mind and body. You cannot think straight or function properly and it can easily trigger depression. Imagine this on top of a difficult birth, a body that needs to recover, worries of a new baby and anger about what has happened… It's the perfect recipe for postnatal depression. It took me about six months to get over the experience and I had to have my second child in a different hospital because I couldn't bear to return there to those memories. You might think I was being overdramatic but I assure you, sleep deprivation does awful things to you.

To think that there are parents out there experiencing the nasty effects of sleep deprivation, perhaps caused by a little one keeping them awake more than necessary, fills me with compassion and leaves me bursting to help because I know, first hand both how terrible it can be when you are suffering and how wonderful it can be when your family is well-rested.

Is This Book For You?

With so many baby sleep books on the shelf, how do you know this is the one for you? Perhaps you have identified that this book is different because it shows you how to figure out the most suitable solutions for YOUR family rather than telling you how to implement one particular method or approach.

By choosing this book, you have already demonstrated that you recognise you have some difficulties that you are keen to resolve. That's an excellent first step.

The next step is to ask yourself the following questions:

- *What would happen if you were to do nothing about your situation and leave everything as it is?*
  - Would your or your family's health suffer?
  - Would your or your family's safety be at risk?
  - Would you continue to suffer rather than enjoy this time?
  - Would your relationship suffer stress and damage?

- *In an ideal world, how would this subject look for you?*
  - Your child going to bed happily?
  - Having some evening time with your partner?
  - Feeling rested and refreshed when you wake up each morning?
  - More patience and more enjoyment with your child during the day?
  - Able to plan around a more predictable sleep schedule?

- *Are you open-minded and willing to look at different options*
  - If your mind is made up that you cannot be helped then you will not be helped.
  - If you believe there is only one way, you will already be doing it.

- *Are you prepared to make changes and commit to them?*
  - If everything stays the same, nothing will change.
  - You'll learn a lot from reading this book but you must actually implement measures in order to see a change.
  - Commitment and consistency are everything.

Get involved in our support community:

We have an online community called The Sleep Centre where other parents who have gone or are going through similar things to you, come together to support each other and share experiences. If you would like to add extra value to this book, join us in The Sleep Centre where we regularly discuss topics from this book. **www.facebook.com/groups/sleepcentre.**

I wanted to keep this book manageable and digestible for tired and busy parents so that it does not just end up on the shelf collecting dust but instead, becomes your guide. The book alone will not make your situation better, but by learning *how* to create the best plan for your family, YOU can.

Secure Attachment

Creating a secure attachment for our children is very important but sometimes this can be confused with attachment parenting or attachment theory which dates back to scientific research in the 1950s. I feel it is important to discuss this topic and to consider all parenting choices because you can teach your child excellent sleep skills regardless of your parenting philosophy.

A secure attachment means that your child feels loved, protected, nurtured and safe in his relationship with you. It is the basis of a child's healthy social, emotional, cognitive and motor development for a baby right through to adulthood. So how do we achieve this?

There are books and theories out there that talk about how to be loving and attentive parents but they also leave parents confused, concerned and feeling guilty that they may be somehow harming their baby by 'doing it wrong' if they choose not to co-sleep or if they choose to teach their baby how to sleep well and independently.

You will achieve a very healthy attachment with your child if you don't try to be perfect (see the chapter on Imperfect Parenting on page 117) and you know that you are 'good enough' at providing that natural love, care, warmth and protection.

When you allow your baby to explore, firstly just across the room and later, running in the park, you are there with reassuring eyes on them, allowing them to be curious and learn with a strong sense of trust between you and your child. It is your role to protect but not wrap them in cotton wool. When they fall over, you are there to wipe away the tears, give comfort and clean up any scratches, allowing them to assess risk and caution in a safe environment under your supervision. Setting clear, consistent and age-appropriate boundaries such as allowing your child to walk ahead of you but just to the next lamp post, gives him a sense of independence. Allowing your child to choose which pyjamas to wear offers choice but within the boundaries of bedtime which is not his choice.

Studies show that the most emotionally stable children are those who have a balance of security and support from their responsive parents along with their own confidence and sense of freedom.

Children need to learn how to deal with emotions such as frustration, anger and excitement and this comes from being able to regulate themselves as we cannot always 'fix' these emotions for them. With sleep, the frustration comes when a baby does not know how to fall asleep, even though it is what she wants to do. If it has always been done for her through rocking or feeding etc... this will be the only way she knows how to get to sleep. My approach to sleep coaching is with a secure attachment, letting them explore how to fall asleep but without leaving them to it and just shutting the door. After the newborn stage, you can practise gentle techniques to shape your baby's ability to learn how to fall asleep and then beyond 18 weeks, you can teach him kindly, gently and supportively to help him to master this life skill while feeling secure that you are always nearby.

Why can't we just keep doing it for them? Because the ability to put oneself to sleep is a learned skill, which means it has to be taught in some way. Just like you feed your baby until she learns how to use the spoon and do it for herself. She learns this through watching you and others do it. Many parents teach their little ones to sleep without even realising they have done any 'teaching' and usually these are cases where the child happens to have an easy temperament and be quite adaptable and the parent's instincts and parenting style, happen to fit nicely with their child's personality.

Sleep Nanny Note:

- Be present when you are with your child.
- Offer comfort and reassurance.
- Allow your child to explore and learn.
- Offer choice within safe boundaries.

The Science Behind Sleep

To understand what is going on with your child, it helps to understand the science. Now, I'm not about to put on a lab coat and bore you with a geeky lesson here but these are some interesting facts that will help make sense of things...

Circadian Rhythms:
Our bodies are programmed to work with nature to establish a body clock and tune in to night and day. These are called circadian rhythms and they are literally learned by natural daylight and darkness. When it is light outside, our brain tells our body that we should be awake and when it is dark we start to get ready for sleep. Babies will naturally develop their circadian rhythms too but it is helpful to give them a nudge in the right direction, especially when we have light evenings/bedtimes and early mornings during the summer months and dark afternoons and mornings in the winter; quite confusing for a little, developing brain.

To encourage your baby to learn night and day you can start off by using blackout blinds and curtains to black out all the natural light in their room. It is okay to use a dim night light, as artificial light doesn't have the same effect on circadian rhythms. It's also a great idea to show other clear signals of night and day whenever you go into your child's room, such as being very quiet and whispering for night-time and being more jolly and energised for daytime.

Sleep Cycles:
We all go though sleep cycles when we sleep. Adult sleep cycles are longer than a baby's and we don't even notice them much of the time. You might just roll over or adjust your pillow and nod back off

without really being very aware that it has happened. At the end of each sleep cycle, comes a partial arousal and most young babies have no idea how to put themselves back to sleep so they become more awake in this partial arousal and then get stuck awake, so they cry for help. Usually this cry is saying, 'help me and do that thing you did that got me to sleep before' which might have been feeding, rocking, holding, stroking... A baby's sleep cycles are roughly 40-60 minutes long. Some babies wake after every sleep cycle and some can manage a longer stretch at a certain time of night and just wake at the end of some of their sleep cycles.

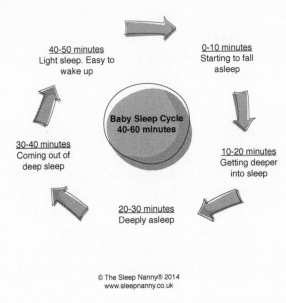

40-50 minutes
Light sleep. Easy to
wake up

0-10 minutes
Starting to fall
asleep

Baby Sleep Cycle
40-60 minutes

30-40 minutes
Coming out of
deep sleep

10-20 minutes
Getting deeper
into sleep

20-30 minutes
Deeply asleep

© The Sleep Nanny® 2014
www.sleepnanny.co.uk

The key is for your baby to be able to resettle back to sleep after each partial arousal without needing your help. It will become so natural to him that he will hardly even know he is doing it.

Being able to settle to sleep and resettle back to sleep is a learned skill and not something we just know how to do like breathing and eating. Learning to self settle is something a baby needs you to teach them but this does not mean you have to leave them to cry and figure it out for themselves. You can actually teach them and show them in a kind and comforting way that is suitable for your child.

Sleep Nanny Note:

- Natural light affects our body clocks.
- We all go through cycles of deeper and lighter states of sleep.
- The ability to put oneself to sleep is a learned skill.
- Once a child can self settle, she will be able to transition from one sleep cycle to the next.

Newborn Sleep

When our newborn first arrives, we have health care providers to help us with how to hold them, feed them, change them, bath them and even swaddle them but they don't tell us how to get them to sleep or even what we should realistically expect from the baby in terms of sleep. We are left with the assumption that it will just fall into place and a baby will just sleep when he needs to. Nobody tells us that it is actually a learned skill. For generations before ours, mothers often stayed at home to raise the children so it didn't matter if they spent hours out walking with a pram or rocking a baby in arms or doing whatever it took to soothe the baby to sleep. This is instinctive as a mother too so it is only natural to want to soothe and comfort your baby.

The modern world we live in today sees more and more working mums raising families and juggling more than women have ever done before. Therefore it is important that we teach our babies how to fall asleep, rather than do it for them, while still being there to comfort them and respond to them as a mother is naturally compelled to.

In the very beginning, the first few weeks, you just need to focus on recovering and bonding with your new baby, learning to feed and enjoying this precious time, not worrying about any kind of schedule or starting any bad habits because you can do no wrong in these early weeks. Newborns do tend to sleep a lot but it is a light slumber rather than a deep sleep. Nevertheless, use this time to get as much rest as you can. They say 'sleep when baby sleeps' and this might be the only time to really do that so grab all the sleep you can and allow others to help you with the housework, cooking and caring for any other children if possible.

Go with your natural instincts and your baby's cues to soothe and comfort him which might include rocking, holding, snuggling in a sling, swinging etc... but once you reach around three weeks, it is helpful to start trying some of the foundation techniques below and establishing some patterns.

Whilst it is not possible to sleep train a baby this young, you can still introduce these foundation techniques to lay the groundwork and shape your little one's sleep to increase his ability to be able to sleep through the night once he is ready developmentally. Your goal now is to help them to develop self-soothing strategies which they can control (not something they need you for such as rocking them or replacing a dummy) - See Sleep Crutches on page 43.

Foundation Techniques:

1. Flexible Routine
You can encourage your baby to understand night and day right from the start and it is never too early to start a bedtime routine. Create a calming process leading up to bedtime to let your baby know what is coming and that this sleep time is different from all the other naps in the daytime. When your baby wakes to start her day, open the curtains, turn on the lights and say 'good morning' in a full voice or sing morning songs – I call this 'dramatic wake-up' because it is a different response than you give at all other waking times in the night and tells your baby that it is now morning time and time to start the day. These signals encourage the development of circadian rhythms – our internal 'body' clock.

One of the most common things young babies come to rely on in order to fall asleep is breastfeeding so it is worth keeping in mind that you will try not to feed your baby to sleep. Don't worry if it cannot be helped sometimes, just try to put him down without feeding to sleep at least once per day for practise. Also try feeding your baby when he wakes up from naps rather at the onset of a nap. A flexible pattern of waking, feeding, playing and sleeping works really well, as the late Tracy Hogg describes it, EASY:

E – eat
A – activity
S – sleep
Y – 'you time'

Feeding on demand is recommended and of course you should feed a hungry baby but understanding when your baby is actually hungry can be much more challenging than it sounds. Sometimes a baby may cry due to the frustration of not being able to get to sleep and offering a feed at every cry can create a feed-to-sleep association. It can also create a pattern of a baby who feeds little and often or 'snacking' as we call it. This makes them not hungry enough to take a full feed but needing to 'top-up' all the time and really disturbs their ability to sleep. Try to distinguish the hungry cries from other cries by trying different solutions before offering a feed.

2. Introduce some soothing techniques

Until your baby finds his own ways to soothe himself, he will need some help from you. Dr Harvey Karp's five 'S's are excellent for newborns:

- Swaddling
- Side holding
- Shh-ing
- Sucking
- Swinging

Watching Dr Harvey Karp perform these five S's with fussing newborns is fascinating. You see the babies go from crying hard and really unsettled to completely calm and content in seconds! These are useful for the first few months to help a baby get to sleep but after this time I advise using them just to calm your baby and not to have her fall asleep doing them. From around the second or third month picking your baby up to soothe and calm and then placing him back down to soothe him within his own cot or sleep space gives him the opportunity to practise settling in the place we want him to sleep. You can pick up, calm and put down your baby as many times as it takes but I find, if it causes him to ramp up the crying even more, it can sometimes be better to make the pick ups less frequent and offer more 'in cot' soothing instead. It may not feel like it is having any affect for some weeks but this practise will be teaching your baby so much and will help him to develop his settling skills in time, when he is more ready.

3. Create an environment conducive to sleep

The environment a baby sleeps in can affect the quality of sleep so making it a quiet, calm and dark place will be a great start. Blacking out all natural light will help to avoid confusing the body clock and your baby wanting to wake with the daylight. If you do need some light, use a low wattage night light, preferably amber colour which is more conducive to sleep. White noise and soothing repetitive sounds can help to drown out a noisy street or household and avoid having anything visually stimulating in the room such as a mobile or light projector as these just encourage your baby to stay awake.

Avoid using the cot as a place to play. Other than for a few minutes upon waking, the cot should be reserved for sleep. Try to put your baby in his cot, Moses basket or crib for at least one of his daytime sleeps even if other naps take place in the pram. The thing with motion sleep is it keeps a baby in a lighter state of sleep so the quality of sleep is not so good. Parents often think their baby has the ability to settle himself to sleep because he does so in the pushchair but don't be fooled by this. It is the motion that soothed him off to sleep just as you will have found yourself feel sleepy or maybe nodding off in a car or train for example. It is better for your baby to have motion sleep than no sleep at all but non-motion sleep and better still, sleep in his own cot, will bring about better quality and possibly quantity of sleep too.

4. Offer a dummy as a soother

Sucking is a natural reflex and a comfort to babies and the latest research suggests that a dummy can serve as protection against SIDS (sudden infant death syndrome). These guidelines are always changing so do check the latest advice. Babies enjoy sucking even when they are not interested in feeding so the option of a dummy or pacifier can fulfil that need without offering an unnecessary feed. If your baby is in fact hungry, she will not be soothed by the dummy. It is recommended to wait until breastfeeding is fully established before offering a dummy to a breastfed baby but a bottle-fed baby can have one sooner. Try not to replace the dummy every time it falls out. Maybe your baby wanted a break from it or is looking for something else to have, hold or do. If you constantly replace it each time it falls out, it will be hard to know what your baby really wants. If she repeatedly disregards it, you'll know for sure that she is looking for something else or some other need to be met. Have a think about continued dummy use once your baby is around six months old. She is likely to gradually become more and more attached to it from this age onwards (see Ditching the Dummy page 57).

5. Practise putting your baby down awake but ready for sleep

If you always put your baby into his cot asleep he will not be aware of where he is or how he got there when he wakes. As he rouses from a sleep cycle, he will feel confused and not know how to get back to sleep because the only way he knows is having you do it for him. This will result in crying out for you to come and help him and could happen throughout the night. Practicing putting him down more awake will give him more awareness of what is happening and where he is and give him the opportunity to settle in his cot, with your help if need be. People often refer to this state as 'drowsy but awake' but this can lead to some confusion as to how drowsy and if the baby goes into his cot too drowsy, he might seem awake, but he will actually be so sleepy that he doesn't knowingly do any self settling because all the settling work was already done for him. I used the word practicing in this section because this really is just something to practise at bedtime or once per day in the early months. Once your baby reaches 18 weeks, you can make this routine rather than just practise and actually give your baby a chance to settle himself.

6. Think through before co-sleeping

Some people enjoy co-sleeping, others end up doing it against their desire and some parents never allow their baby into their bed. It is a personal choice and neither one is right or wrong. As long as co-sleeping is done safely and it is serving a purpose then, enjoy. Many parents come to me asking how they can end co-sleeping because it is not for them and I see it used as a 'quick fix' solution at 5 a.m. all the time!

Right from the start, it is a great idea to have a think about this and decide how you and your partner feel about it because once a baby gets used to co-sleeping it is very rare they voluntarily give it up and you will need to consider a transitional process at some stage, to keep your child in her own bed. Whatever you decide be consistent with the message you are sending your child. It is either okay or it is not okay to sleep in your bed. If you allow it once or only after 5 a.m., your child will cry and hold out for this result any time he chooses because he does not understand your reasons as to when it is and is not okay or what 'time' even means!

Between 3-6 months or when your child is ready for his own room, it is wise to transition out of co-sleeping if you are ready.

Sleep Nanny Note:

- Newborn sleep is often very disorganised and naps can take three to five months to become more structured.
- Do not worry about creating 'bad habits' as these can easily be undone at around four to six months of age.
- Start a simple bedtime routine at as early as one to two weeks.
- Create a sleep friendly environment.
- Introduce some soothing techniques to comfort your baby as she attempts to settle to sleep in her own sleep space.

Identifying Your Child's Temperament

Temperament traits determine personality and play a huge part in figuring out the right sleep solution for your child, but how do you know what kind of temperament your child really has? It might be easy to recognise traits such as, strong-willed or sociable but what do these traits mean for your little one's sleep?

Temperament is a set of traits that a child is born with. They help to determine personality and therefore, behaviour. Each temperament will show a different behavioural style or manner in which a child interacts with the environment. Let's take a look at the nine temperament traits:

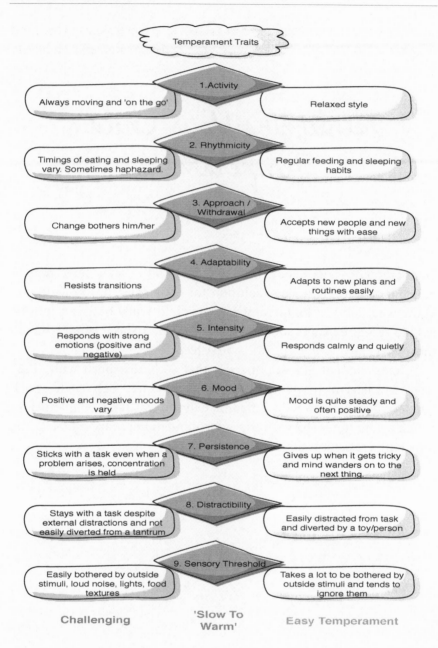

Temperament Traits

1. Activity
Always moving and 'on the go' | Relaxed style

2. Rhythmicity
Timings of eating and sleeping vary. Sometimes haphazard. | Regular feeding and sleeping habits

3. Approach / Withdrawal
Change bothers him/her | Accepts new people and new things with ease

4. Adaptability
Resists transitions | Adapts to new plans and routines easily

5. Intensity
Responds with strong emotions (positive and negative) | Responds calmly and quietly

6. Mood
Positive and negative moods vary | Mood is quite steady and often positive

7. Persistence
Sticks with a task even when a problem arises, concentration is held | Gives up when it gets tricky and mind wanders on to the next thing.

8. Distractibility
Stays with a task despite external distractions and not easily diverted from a tantrum | Easily distracted from task and diverted by a toy/person

9. Sensory Threshold
Easily bothered by outside stimuli, loud noise, lights, food textures | Takes a lot to be bothered by outside stimuli and tends to ignore them

Challenging | 'Slow To Warm' | Easy Temperament

The temperament traits in a child will give you clues as to the kind of environment s/he is most comfortable in. For example, adaptability measures how easily a child can adjust to a change in circumstances or routine. A more adaptable baby will be more likely to sleep better at night.

Alert babies are very active, wilful, determined, prone to temper tantrums, take everything in and they need stronger boundaries. They have a difficult time handling their emotions.

An easy baby is easy-going, adapts well to new situations, is social, reaches milestones on cue, easy to calm, very portable and tends to fall into a natural schedule.

A slow to warm baby is sensitive, shy, prefers order and predictability, is thoughtful and cautious and can become very engrossed in an activity and get frustrated if not allowed to finish it. These children weigh things up carefully and will usually suss someone out before willingly going to them.

A fussy baby needs things his way, can be obstinate, easily frustrated, prefers his own company, will cry as though it is the end of the world, is insightful, resourceful, wise and creative.

A high needs baby is intense, draining, demanding, unsatisfied, unpredictable, supersensitive, extremely active and needs constant attention. They are quick to protest change, can be squirmy and they prefer people to things. This temperament can be a challenge.

Super alert children often show characteristics of the alert babies, slow to warm and fussy babies as described above. They can be difficult to manage as babies but this kind of personality can be of huge benefit later on in life (if managed with clear messages, boundaries and consistency).

Generally, children tend to fit one of three pretty broad and loosely defined categories:

- Easy
- Alert (sometimes challenging)
- Slow-To-Warm

Around 40% of children fit the easy-going category but you are likely to be reading this book because your child is more alert and challenging. These children have a harder time shutting down and blocking out the world around them which makes it much harder for them to settle. They also need regularity and rhythmicity of routine more so than an easy baby.

Depending on just how alert and engaging your child is, will determine the most suitable approach to sleep training for them. There is no point embarking upon a plan that has you staying in the room with them while they fall asleep if this is going to be too stimulating for them. Sometimes, it is kinder to actually give them a little space and check on them frequently. More on that to follow.

Sleep Nanny Note:

- Understanding your little one's temperament helps you to select the best approaches for them.
- Alert children often need more sleep than average and hold on to their daytime naps for longer too.
- Create an environment and routine to suit your child's temperament.

Understanding Sleep Training Approaches

It's a common misconception to think that sleep training must mean leaving a child to cry it out or be, in some way, cruel to put a child through sleep training. It doesn't have to be that way at all. The controversy comes from some of the more harsh philosophies of extinction – which means leaving a baby to cry it out, and this is often compared to how young children in orphanages might be treated. Attempting this kind of approach, particularly with a young baby is where the 'bad press' comes from. Firstly, it is not recommended to sleep train a baby under the age of 18 weeks and secondly, it is very important to find the right, gentle approach to suit your child and your parenting style. At no point does sleep training mean crying it out.

There is so much conflicting advice available on child sleep, it's no wonder we are left confused. The Sleep Nanny System™ is an approach tailored to the individual but always based on the two gentle core methods, as there really are only four methods anyway. As you can see in my gentle sleep scale model, they range from the harsh end of the scale with Extinction, better known as Cry It Out to Ferberizing or Controlled Crying. Then we have the approach of Fading which is sometimes referred to as Gradual Retreat and finally Attachment Parenting at the other end of the scale. There are many different slants on these approaches which frequently pop up under a different name but the core principles of each are the same.

Gentle Sleep Scale

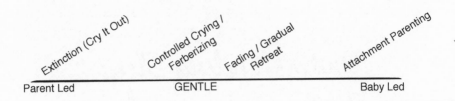

Let's take a closer look at each:

Cry It Out

This is also known as extinction. It is not a method that I advocate because it is not gentle and does not allow you to comfort your child. This method requires you to put your baby down to sleep and leave the room without returning. The idea is that the child will eventually stop crying and learn to fall asleep by himself. There may be some children for whom this is effective but I have never encountered a case that could not be resolved with a more gentle approach.

Key points:
- This is not a method to experiment with. If it's not for you, leave it alone. There is no gain in leaving your child to cry for an extended period of time only to then go in and pick him up and comfort him as this will just teach him to cry harder and for longer.

Pros:
- I don't believe there are any!
- If you are capable of seeing it through, you might expect very fast results.

Cons:
- Not many parents could see this through.
- Studies have shown that babies who are left alone to cry for extended periods of time on a regular basis may be exposed to unhealthy stress levels.

Controlled Crying

This involves leaving your child to try to settle by himself but going back in to offer comfort and reassurance at set intervals. There are many variants of this method which became popular through the Ferberizing technique by Dr Richard Ferber. Some examples of this method suggest you go in every 10 minutes, others have you go in at gradually increasing lengths of time every time for example, after 2 minutes then 4, then 6 then 8 until you reach 10 minutes and then stick to 10. And some examples will increase this up to 15 minute intervals or more. With this method, like any really, you must be 100% consistent so it's wise to get very clear on your planned timings before you start.

Key Points:
- If you set a 10-minute check time, wait the full 10 minutes and don't go in at 9 minutes.
- This is not ideal for a parent who has a zero tolerance for crying.

Pros:
- Highly effective for faster results.
- Still offers comfort and reassurance and not harmful to your child.
- Easily adaptable and mouldable to suit different families.

Cons:
- You will experience some crying whilet not with your baby.
- Can be tough on the caregiver between each check.

Fading

This method is very gentle and involves staying in the room with your child until she falls asleep. You use shh-ing sounds, key phrases or words and intermittent touch, to soothe and comfort your baby. Once she is truly asleep, you leave the room and then return and repeat the same thing for each and every waking until morning. Each night, or every three nights, you should move your position further away from the cot or bed until you are right by the door, then outside the door where she can still see and/or hear you. By the end of this process you should have a child who can put herself to sleep and resettle without needing your help.

Key Points:
- You must be very 'boring' and not interact with your child while you are in the room.
- Any touch should be intermittent, otherwise it may become relied upon.
- Stay put until she is asleep. If you leave too soon, you'll lose the trust and have to start over.
- This is an ideal approach if you have a sleep crutch to eliminate.

Pros:
- Very gentle.
- You can stay with your baby.
- Can be modified for a child in a bed.

Cons:
- Babies can be too stimulated by you.
- Requires one caregiver to be available to spend a lot of time in the room.

Attachment Parenting

As explained in the chapter 'Secure Attachment' it is important for your baby to feel loved, safe and secure. However the approach of attachment parenting takes this to extremes in that it does not allow your baby to learn, explore and make mistakes.

When using attachment parenting as an approach to sleep this would involve co-sleeping or room sharing for as long as the baby wants, baby wearing or using a sling for most naps, settling your baby with whatever works be it rocking, cuddling, feeding, stroking and generally responding to your baby in a 'rescue' sense every time she fusses. Feeding on demand is fine, particularly during the early months but using feeding as a means to settle a baby even when they are not hungry, is not truly serving him.

Attachment parenting techniques are valuable for newborns but it is wise to look at the long-term effects too. You should also consider who you are doing this for, you or your baby. Some parents feel that, whilst it is tiring for them, it seems best for their baby, while others might reach a point where they notice it is not really benefiting their baby but they enjoy all the cuddles and don't feel ready to move on.

Pros:
- Path of least resistance.
- Easy to implement.
- Lots of cuddles to enjoy.

Cons:
- A child will not end this through choice for many years.
- The longer you use this approach, the harder it is to teach your child to sleep independently.
- Might make life easy in the short term but can make things tougher in the long term.
- Your child may lack vital skills and this could reflect in other behaviour too.

At each end of the spectrum are approaches I do not teach. One (Extinction) is very harsh and unresponsive which I do not advocate and the other (attachment parenting) is a lifestyle choice that works for people who are not looking for assistance in teaching their child essential independent sleep skills at this time. Therefore, it is within the two middle, gentle approaches that I base my philosophies and trainings. I call these Regulated Responding and Four-Step Fade-Out.

My recommendation is to do what feels right for your family and respond to your child but, by 4-6 months, it will be beneficial to introduce a gentle and responsive approach to sleep because your baby will learn such valuable and essential life skills such as self-regulation.

No parent deliberately wants to upset their child or put them through any stress or fear. This is why I am a big proponent of gentle methods. Being a mother myself, I know how difficult it is to see your child upset. Some dads are the same but quite often the dads are more resilient than the mums. It is the way we are wired. Nature makes our babies' cries pull on our heartstrings. It is our instinct to comfort our children and why shouldn't you?

There is no point in choosing a sleep training plan that involves controlled crying for example, if you cannot bear to leave your child for even just a few minutes. It will not be effective if you cannot see it through so be sure you choose a plan that you can be totally consistent with.

Many mothers require a sleep training approach that allows them to comfort their baby and respond to his cries. This is where the gentle philosophy comes in; being with your child as she learns how to put herself to sleep, offering a comforting touch or voice to reassure her that you are there. This works very well but, in some cases, it is just not best suited to the child's temperament. Should the parent persist with what is right for themselves or be strong and go with an approach that better suits the child even though it is not easy for the parent? Well, you are likely to see faster results by working to your child's needs but only if you stick to it so, to make this more comfortable for you, tweak the method to make it suitable for both the child's temperament and the parenting style. This is what I do for families every day. Create bespoke training plans.

For example, let's say your child is far too stimulated by having you in the room with them. He tries to play with you or chat to you or wants to interact with you. He simply cannot leave you alone and just take comfort in your presence. This might mean you need to leave him for periods of between 5-15 minutes and keep returning to calm him, reassure him and step out again. If it is too tough for you to leave him for even five minutes, then you might need to modify this approach with the end stages of a more gentle approach. When you leave the room, instead of going downstairs and burying your head under a cushion until the next check, you could sit just outside his room with the door ajar and reassure him with shh-ing sounds so that he knows you are nearby. This is just one example of modifying an approach to make it work for you.

Looking at these examples, you can see how different temperaments might respond. For example, a baby who does not like change or is very attached to being held or rocked to sleep will be well suited to the Four-Step Fade-Out method to gently transition him from this, to being able to settle himself to sleep. However, if the child is very easily stimulated by the presence of people, he may do better with Regulated Responding and being left alone for short periods to give him a chance to settle himself without the distraction of a parent in the room.

Finding the right balance between what feels right for you as a parent and what suits your child will be your first step to creating a really effective solution. One you can follow through with total consistency and that your child can progress and learn independent sleep skills from.

Selecting Your Gentle Sleep Training Approach

Four-Step Fade Out:

This works really well if there is an obvious sleep crutch that you want to wean your baby off. Quite often the sleep crutch is you or at least associated with you or you doing something, so this approach slowly weans the need for you to 'do it for your child' and offers a nice support and reassurance level if you have removed an object such as a dummy or a feed to sleep association, for example.

How it works:

Night one you sit in a chair right next to the cot or bed until she falls asleep. You're not there to interact and it's better if you can be as boring as possible in your body language. You can pat or shh intermittently for comfort but make sure it is intermittent and not constantly until she is asleep, otherwise this is just a new sleep crutch in the making. If she becomes hysterical, you can pick her up to clam her down and then place her straight back down. Just pick up to calm and as soon as she is calm, which might be right away, she needs to go back down. Yes, she will cry when she goes back down and you might have to repeat the process after more trying at the other soothing techniques. If picking her up makes her more angry, it might be kinder to just soothe her in the cot rather than pick her up.

You stay in the room in the same spot, until she is asleep. It might take some time but that first night, when she puts herself to sleep, she has made a massive leap in learning. Do the same for two more nights and then on the fourth night, move your chair halfway between the cot and the door and continue the process in this position for three nights. After that, move your chair position to just inside the door for three nights and then move outside the room but so she can still hear you for three nights.

These are the four steps to the process:

Step one: you are next to the cot.

Step two: you are halfway between the cot and the furthest point away in the room.

Step three: you are as far away from the cot as you can be while still in the room and in view.

Step four: you are outside of the room but can still be heard.

Every night, your aim is to reduce how much soothing help you give. Think of it in three stages of necessity:

Stage one: You just need to be present in the room, in view.

Stage two: You need to be present and heard with some soothing shh-ing sounds or whispering keywords.

Stage three: This requires the presence, the sounds and the touch with patting or stroking for reassurance.

At first you will use all three but gradually reduce each night until just being there is enough.

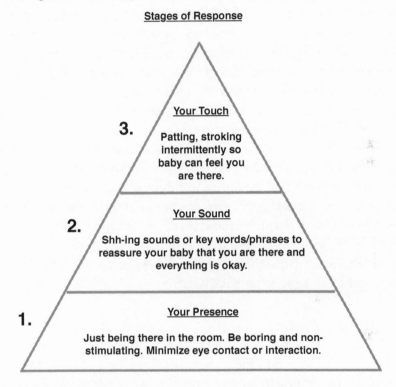

Stages of Response

3. Your Touch — Patting, stroking intermittently so baby can feel you are there.

2. Your Sound — Shh-ing sounds or key words/phrases to reassure your baby that you are there and everything is okay.

1. Your Presence — Just being there in the room. Be boring and non-stimulating. Minimize eye contact or interaction.

Pyramid of Parental Help © 2015 The Sleep Nanny®

When your child wakes during the night, it's important to respond in the same way every time and this should match what you did at bedtime. So matching your position from bedtime, you need to go in and sit in your current position for any waking in the night and stay there until she is back to sleep.

Wake-up Time

Set a time that you'll call wake-up time. No earlier than 6 a.m., somewhere between 6-7 a.m. usually works well, and then treat anything before this time as a night waking and respond accordingly. If, for example, you have 6 a.m. as wake-up time and she wakes up at 5.40 a.m. and you go in and take up your position, and she doesn't resettle before wake-up time and you are still there in the room, don't just go from sitting there, to getting her up because this will tell her that if she holds out long enough, eventually you'll just give in and take her out of the cot. Instead you need to use a 'dramatic wake-up' to signify the difference between night and day. The best way to do this is to step out of the room for a minute, I mean a whole 60 seconds, even if there is yelling, and then go back in all bright and breezy turning on the lights or opening the curtains. We want to show the difference between how you enter the room to respond to a night waking – all zombielike, boring and quiet, and how you enter the room to get her up in the morning, vocal, jolly and bright. Practicing 'dramatic wake-up' every day, even when you didn't find yourself stuck in the room, will start to teach your child to immediately recognise whether it is time to get up or time to go back to sleep.

Regulated Responding:

The Four-Step Fade-Out might be too stimulating if your child is not used to having you in their room. They might try to play with you or think you are going to get them up because normally you leave the room. I do recommend giving it a go for three to five nights anyway, especially if there is an obvious sleep crutch which they will be missing from you. However, you may have to try using Regulated Responding if it causes too much stimulation to be in the room.

You do your goodnight routine, say night-night and leave the room. Your baby might call for you, cry or scream but you can go back to check on her after a pre-decided number of minutes. Somewhere between every 5-15 minutes, depending on what you are comfortable with. I can tell you, the longer you can go between checks, the more quickly this works. If in doubt, go for 10 minute checks – they work wonders.

Every time you respond, go into the room in 'boring' mode (you're not there to rescue her or to interact) and start by just shh-ing and/or whisper keywords such as 'lie down' or 'sleepy time'. If you need to add some touch, that's fine but try to keep your baby in the cot and only pick her up if she is really hysterical. If you do pick up – just pick up to calm her down and as soon as she is calm, put her back down. Be brief in your visit. No more than 30 seconds in the room before you leave again and wait for enough time to pass before the next check. Repeat this process for as long as it takes for your little one to put herself to sleep.

This technique offers the reassurance that you are still nearby and will always return but also sends the message that it is now time to lie down and go to sleep and it gives your child the opportunity to practise putting herself to sleep.

Whatever you decide is right for you, be sure to stick to it and not chop and change and send mixed messages. You're either in the room for the long haul or you're not. Don't stay for a while using the Four-Step Fade Out plan and then leave because you got fed up and decided to see if she would settle if you left her for 10 minutes. This is confusing and takes away that reassurance we are trying to give.

Sleep Nanny Note:

- Use your understanding of your child's temperament to select the most suitable sleep training approach for them.
- There are only four main categories for sleep training methods.
- Be clear, confident and prepared before you start.
- Only commence if you are committed to seeing it through, otherwise you could confuse your child and be worse off than before.
- Remember, consistency is KEY.

Routine

Humans are creatures of habit and children thrive on routine. A routine gives signals to a baby or young child as to what is coming next. For example, it is bath time so bedtime is approaching. When I talk about routine, I always tell families to do the same things, in the same order every time. This lets your child know what to expect, helps them to feel secure as it is all familiar and sets clear boundaries as to what is and is not appropriate for this time of day.

Keeping a structured bedtime routine will prevent things like a preschooler asking to go outside to play after bath time. Okay, so they might ask because let's face it, they will try all sorts at that age but they will know that this is not actually an option if they have a routine in place where bath time is followed by bedtime.

Do you have a suitable bedtime routine in place already? Most young children do well with a bedtime between the hours of 6 and 8 p.m. and you'll want around 30-40 minutes of routine to lead up to that bedtime. It's ideal to turn off the TV and any screens for a few hours before bedtime but if this is a struggle, at least try to have a bit of activity time without the TV on as the last thing they do before the bedtime routine starts. Many people start the bedtime routine with a bath and that is a great way to send the signals that bedtime is getting close because it is something totally different to anything else you do in the day. Some children do get very playful and lively in the bath and that's fine, the bath is actually quite calming even though a child might appear very active while in the bath. This might be followed by a nice low-key and calm process of getting dry and dressed, brushing teeth and going into the room that they'll be sleeping in and then a bedtime story or that last feed of the day, or whatever you usually do next. Just be sure to do the same steps in the same order every night. If your little one falls asleep on a feed at bedtime, it's a good idea to introduce a step after the feed, like a book to look at or a nursery rhyme, something to stay awake for.

Sleep Nanny Note:

- Routines act as a series of cues that tell your little one what is happening.
- Rhythm is formed from routine and helps little ones feel secure.
- Routines help the body naturally prepare for sleep and wakeful times.

Sleep Crutches

I'm sure you have heard the term 'sleep crutch' before. Or perhaps 'prop' or 'sleep association'? They all mean the same thing, that they refer to something your baby relies on in order to get to sleep.

The difference between a sleep association, to a prop or a crutch, is that a sleep association can be positive or negative while a prop or crutch tend to be negative. Let me explain...

If your baby has a sleep association such as a particular soft toy that he likes to take to bed, that is positive because it is something he can control. However, if your child has a sleep association of being rocked to sleep by you, this is negative because he needs you to do it for him and has no control over this himself.

Is a dummy a sleep crutch?

The dummy has its own set of rules depending on how it is used. If your child has control of the dummy or does not need you to replace it at any point if it falls out, then this might not be a problem but it is still a sleep association if he requires it to fall asleep.

On the other hand, if your baby needs you to keep re-plugging the dummy every time it falls out and cannot resettle without you coming to do this, then it is a sleep crutch that is not helping.

Sleep crutches can be all sorts of things but the most common ones are, feeding to sleep, rocking, patting, holding and co-sleeping. None of these are a big problem in the early months and you cannot spoil a newborn so don't panic if your young baby needs this kind of help from you for now but you do need a plan to remove these crutches by the age of around six months if you don't want to continue this way for the next few years!

It is reasonably easy to remove a sleep crutch around the age of six months when a baby is most adaptable and accepting of change. From this age on, the longer you leave it, the more difficult it is likely to become because the habits will become more ingrained and your child will be more resistant to change.

So now you can identify a sleep crutch and determine whether it is serving a purpose or is a hindrance to your baby's sleep. The next step is to form a plan, either for now or for the coming months, if you need to wean a baby off a sleep crutch.

Sleep Nanny Note:

- A sleep crutch is something your child relies on you to do for them in order for them to fall asleep.
- If your little one relies on a sleep crutch at bedtime, he will be likely to require the same thing to get back to sleep if he wakes in the night.
- Around the age of six months, it is relatively easy to remove a sleep crutch.

Early Risers

Early risers can leave us feeling so tired and can totally mess with a child's nap schedule too. Anything before 6 a.m. is just inhumane right? I had an early riser so I know the pain that comes with this but, once you know the cause and you tackle the problem, you and your child can feel refreshed and start your day at a 'normal' hour! The most common cause of early rising, in a nutshell, is over tiredness.

This can come in the form of these four top causes:
1. Too late a bedtime.
2. Nap deprivation.
3. Too much time between the afternoon nap and bedtime.
4. Putting the child to bed when they're too sleepy at bedtime.

In many cases the child does not get enough sleep during the day. Parents often underestimate how much sleep their child really needs and fall into the trap of thinking they are not sleepy by bedtime which leads them to keeping them up too late. In actual fact, children often appear to be wide awake at bedtime when they are actually overtired. When a sleep window is missed, the brain thinks 'the lights are still on, there's lots going on, I need to wake up!' and hormones are released, such as cortisol which is like a shot of adrenaline. This will 'wire' your child and give off the illusion that they are far too awake to go to sleep. The longer you keep them up, the more cortisol is released and the tougher it becomes to settle them.

Do not be fooled by those alert little ones either. They are very good at hiding their sleepy signs and you really need to keep an eye on the clock with these guys. Know what the average sleep requirements are for your child's age and use them as a close guide. Also, be aware of the average wakeful windows for their age – how long a stretch they can go between sleeps. This might not be as long as your child would have you think!

Many parents allow their child to drop their nap altogether around the age of two and a half to three years. This can often be due to fitting in with the day care routine or it can be parents feeling that their child no longer needs the nap. If you drop the nap and then find a few months down the line that you have an early riser or he struggles to settle at bedtime or he is up and down all night – the chances are he really does still need that nap.

Often babies in the six to twelve month bracket and possibly more so in the nine to twelve month section when they are on a two-nap schedule, are not at their best in the late afternoon. If the gap between the afternoon nap and bedtime is too large, the child gets overtired and the 'stay awake' hormone, cortisol gets in the way. To avoid this, an emergency catnap of up to 30 minutes can really do the trick. This can be as late as about 4 p.m. as long as the child is awake by 4.30 p.m. and that is based on bedtime being at about 7 p.m.

Finally, one of my top tips for keeping your toddler in bed until morning is to introduce a day/night clock. There are many variations out there but it needs to be very simple and clear for your toddler to understand. My favourite is one that simply shows a rabbit in bed when your child should be in bed and when rabbit wakes up, your child is allowed to get up. Children can grasp this from around 21 months but you can introduce the clock sooner so they can start to get familiar with it. The golden rule with this one is: NEVER get your child up or allow them to start their day before 'rabbit is up'. If you do, they will never take the clock seriously again.

Overcoming early rising is the best feeling in the world. Not only do you get the full night's sleep you need without having to sacrifice your evening and go to bed at the same time as your child but also your child benefits greatly from the sleep too. Your baby's routine and nap schedule will work better if she doesn't start her day too early and sleep is vital to child brain development too, so fixing an issue like early rising really is a must for all the family.

Sleep Nanny Note:

- Early rising is most commonly caused by over tiredness.
- Early rising can take several weeks to resolve.
- If your child wakes up crying or miserable this is a sign that he has not had enough sleep.
- Special day/night clocks are a good aid to a training plan to help an early rising toddler.
- It is important to change the environment when your child gets up for the day to clearly mark the difference between day and night. No slumber in the parents' room.

Case Study: Thomas aged two years and three months.

When Thomas' parents contacted me, Thomas was taking more than an hour to settle at bedtime, waking frequently in the night and starting his day between 5.30 a.m. and 6 a.m. each morning. He was no longer in a cot but had his own bed in his own room. Frequently he would go through to his parents' room in the night and climb into bed with them where he would not really sleep particularly well but it was the only way the parents could get any sleep. Thomas would take a varying length nap in the day some days either on the sofa or on the go.

It was clear to me that Thomas was a very alert little boy, he had reached several developmental milestones earlier than average and could hold quite an advanced conversation for his age. His parents had been very attentive and this inquisitive little boy would insist on constant interaction with them. Needless to say, at bedtime, he was not keen to be left alone in his room to go to sleep and would engage in as much interaction with his parents as he could.

Due to the attachment I could see Thomas had to having someone with him to help him fall asleep, I knew we would need to gradually help him learn to fall asleep on his own, starting off with a parent staying with him by his side and, over the course of 10-14 nights, working on reducing the parent's assistance until no longer required.

My main concern about this approach for this little boy was that he was so alert and would definitely try his hardest to interact with his parents making them an added stimulation in the room. When being in the room is too stimulating, I would recommend the Regulated Responding approach from outside the room only making very brief visits of reassurance and calming because some little ones do better when given a little space. However, I did not think Thomas was ready to let go of his parents being beside him just yet and neither were the parents so we took things very gently.

Thomas went through his bedtime routine with no problem and would get into bed for his story but as soon as the lights went out, he came alive. At first, Thomas would get up and literally climb on his parents for attention. He would head towards the door and look back at his parent for a reaction but when he didn't get one, he would return to his bed. The parents had to be like human statues in the room because the slightest interaction would become a game for Thomas. Each night would be the same regardless of how close or how far away his parents sat from his bed but we knew persistence would prevail in the end.

After a week, Thomas began to only get up one or two times at bedtime and then go back and stay in his bed and go to sleep. In the night he would go into his parents' room to be happily guided back to his bed where he would then stay. It was as though he just wanted to involve them in his resettling. By the end of week two he was staying in his bed at bedtime and very rarely coming out in the night but, even when he did, he would quickly resettle once guided back to bed. It took a further 10 days for the morning wake-up to stretch out to 6.30 a.m. and this followed an improvement in daytime naps.

Naps – More on naps and their importance

How well does your baby or toddler nap? Do they seem overtired by the end of the day? Do you find your child will not nap but will fall asleep in the car? Let me tell you a little bit about the importance of naps and the surprising amount of daytime sleep our little ones really need...

So why are naps so important? Firstly, sleep in general supports your child's brain development and is good for their health overall but also, sleep begets sleep and a baby who is nap deprived will become overtired and more likely to:

- Struggle to settle at bedtime (seem wide awake but actually too tired to sleep).
- Have night awakenings.
- Wake too early in the morning and want to start his day (anything before 6 a.m. is too early).

It can sound a bit backwards that a child can be too tired to sleep but I assure you that this is a mistake that so many parents make. 'If my child has a nap during the day, he won't go to sleep at night' – I hear that a lot. The thing is, the child is actually so overtired and nap deprived that his body becomes flooded with cortisol (a natural adrenaline) and his instinct is to fight sleep.

So how much sleep should our children get during the day?
Newborn babies nap a LOT but this sleep is much lighter and very disorganised. Right through to around four months of age, you

might find naps to be very irregular. Around 4-6 months, naps will be able to take more of a schedule so you can teach your baby to take these naps in her cot to get the best quality of sleep and perhaps a little break for you too!

From around four months they will move into a more organised 'three naps per day' routine which will transition to two naps per day somewhere around eight months approximately. Some start to show signs of being ready to drop to one nap as early as 12 months but are not likely to be truly ready just yet. The average age to drop to one nap is 15-17 months and this one nap will start off being about two and a half hours long just after lunch (12/12.30 p.m. is ideal).

I find many parents stop the nap altogether around age two and a half or if their child goes to preschool but this is actually very young to stop napping. 95% of children actually still need some form of daytime nap until age three and a half or even four years!

Making a change to the nap schedule, stopping naps completely or adding one back in, takes a transitional period to take effect. For example, before I became a sleep coach, my eldest stopped napping when he moved up from toddler's nursery to preschool because that's just what everyone else did. It took about three months of his night-time sleep gradually deteriorating and the early rising creeping in before I asked myself why this was happening. As soon as I figured out that this was due to over tiredness, I reintroduced his daytime nap and within a week, his night-time sleep was back on track! If ever the nap was short or missed, I would get him to bed early to compensate and his night-time sleep improved no end.

Once they reach the transitional age where the nap is almost no longer needed, they might nap some days and not other days and then stop napping but occasionally nod off in the car (a sign that they do still need that little bit of sleep in the day). You can help them through the transition with early nights when needed and within a few months, the transitional period will pass. See more about nap transitions on page 53.

A child who naps well is more likely to sleep well at night time so long as the naps are at the right sort of times of day (i.e. not too close to bedtime). Keeping your child awake to try to get them to sleep better at night is a total myth and will have the opposite effect.

Having an understanding of how long your child's wakeful

windows are – that is, how long they can be awake in one stretch before needing another sleep – will hugely help you to find the most ideal nap schedule for them. For example, a new baby will only be able to manage 45 minutes awake before needing to be asleep again so help her back to sleep after that time. An eight-month-old will be able to be awake for about two-three hours per stretch and a 22-month-old will manage around five to five and a half hours before needing to sleep.

So if your child gets irritable during the day, has meltdowns before bedtime or is a little early bird, ask yourself if he is getting enough sleep during the day and going to bed early enough because, remember this phrase, 'sleep begets sleep'.

Let's take a look at the three most common nap training outcomes and what to do about them…

Does not go to sleep at all for an entire hour of trying:

In this instance, do your dramatic wake-up routine, open the curtains and be all jolly and bright and get your child up. If this means he has skipped his morning nap, he won't be able to last until the afternoon for the next nap so watch out for sleepy signs and be ready to try again much sooner that you would have, even if that is in just 45 minutes' time.

The next possible outcome is:

Only naps for 45 minutes; this is the minimum you want to be seeing for the first nap and if he wakes up happy and seems refreshed, that's fine but bear in mind that he might be ready for his second nap sooner, for example, after two hours rather than three, so watch for sleepy signs so that you don't miss the next sleep window. Usually, if a child has woken up happy after just 45 minutes in the morning, he won't wake up happy and refreshed on just 45 minutes for the afternoon nap so if this happens, use the Four-Step Fade-Out approach or Regulated Responding to encourage him back to sleep and try for at least 30 minutes if you can.

So what if he naps for less than 45 minutes?

This is what we call a disaster nap because it tends to just be one sleep cycle and the child hasn't managed to resettle after just one sleep cycle. This is really common, especially when they haven't yet got the self-settling skills mastered so be prepared for a few of these in the early stages of nap coaching. Technically, this wide-eyed state that they wake in is actually a partial arousal and not true wakefulness. So here's what to do and I have to tell you this is tough... You need to go to him and use the Four-Step Fade-Out or Regulated Responding and do it for one hour. This is called the longest hour in my profession. So here's an example... He goes in the cot at 9 a.m. and takes until 9.30 to settle to sleep, then only sleeps until 10 a.m. so you go in and work on getting him back to sleep which he does eventually at 10.40 a.m. but then he only sleeps for a further 20 minutes! Chances are, you'll be thinking 'why did she tell me to do that, he was awake more than he was asleep, what was the point?' Well, the point is that even though it took 40 minutes for him to get back to sleep, he did it! He put himself back to sleep from a partial arousal in a nap and that is a massive achievement. The more he gets used to doing this the sooner he will be able to glide over those partial arousals and take longer naps on his own. You just have to stick with it.

Always have a backup plan. It is so important when nap training because things can be all over the place with timing for a while. Your primary aim is to make sure he is getting enough daytime sleep in total. I recommend trying at least one nap per day in the cot, two if you can but if it has to be a motion nap, this is better than no nap at all. If you try for an hour and he does not go to sleep at all, go to the backup plan of a pushchair nap but to do this, make sure you step out of the room for 60 seconds first and then go back in with a dramatic wake-up. We don't want him to think that if he holds out for an hour you'll just get him up, so we have to make a clear break between trying to get him to go to sleep and going in merrily to get him up because you chose to, not because he's cried hard enough.

Also, if you are on the transition from three naps to two, you may need to use an afternoon 'buggy nap' or catnap as a backup plan for those days when he is feeling more tired or hasn't slept well. You could also opt for an earlier bedtime during any transitional phase or on a day when naps have just been a bit short. 30-60 minutes earlier to bed can actually make all the difference on those days and don't worry, that doesn't mean an earlier start – it doesn't work that way as you now know, right?

Transitioning Naps

When it comes to transitioning from three naps to two, from two naps to one and from one nap to no nap, it is important to be aware of the bumpy phase this might bring.

The transition from three to two is fairly straightforward and usually occurs quite naturally between the ages of seven - nine months. That third nap of the day becomes shorter and less necessary while the morning and afternoon naps stabilise. If your baby is struggling with bedtime and night times, the chances are that naps will be a problem too. Don't worry and work on bedtime first, then night times and finally naps because evidence shows naps are the last piece to fall into place. In the meantime, just aim for the quantity of daytime sleep that is right for your child's age.

The two big transitions with naps are when they go from two to one and from one to none! These transitions can take anything from a couple of weeks to a few months to complete so don't expect an overnight transformation. During this time your child is likely to need more sleep on some days than others.

Transitioning from two naps to one

How do you know when your baby is ready?
This transition typically occurs between the ages of 13-17 months and by 18 months, most babies are taking one afternoon nap. This nap may or may not be the same length as the previous two naps were. Often when they first transition, this one nap is longer and will soon stabilise as they become more adjusted to the change.

The most common signs that your child is ready to transition are:
- Stops taking one of the naps.
- Takes longer and longer to fall asleep for one or both naps.
- Misses morning nap and is fine or doesn't take a longer afternoon nap to compensate.

How to make the transition:
If you are sure your little one is ready, you can either:
- Keep him up all morning and just put him down for an afternoon nap.
- Gradually shift the morning nap later and later in increments of 15-30 minutes every few days while the afternoon nap may become quite short until the two meet in the middle as one nap.
- If your child is not ready to make a big leap or shows signs very early, it may take more time with a mixture of two-nap days and one-nap days. Follow your child's lead in this case.

Remember: An early bedtime is a very useful backup plan for those days when he needs more sleep or just didn't nap so well.

One-nap Routine:
It really helps to create a routine for one nap and this tends to work well for most children right after lunch. Not only are they naturally ready for a sleep by then but it also creates an association that after lunch is nap time. Use a short routine of 5-15 minutes in your child's room to read a book or have a song and wind down in the dark to ease them from the bright activities of the day to the quiet and calm of nap time.

Transitioning from one nap to no nap:
Typically, children are ready to drop the nap altogether somewhere between age three and four years but some still have some daytime sleep right up to age five or even six years! So there's no rush to drop the nap.

How do you know when your child is ready?

The most common signs that your child no longer needs a nap are:
- Stops falling asleep at nap time.
- Takes longer and longer to fall asleep at nap time.
- Does not nap and is fine and not overtired by bedtime.
- Does not nap and stays awake on a late afternoon car ride.

How to make this transition:

It is not likely to happen overnight and your child may need a nap some days and not others. He may even go for a few weeks of not needing to nap in the day and then seem to need one again for a while or on some days. This could be due to activities or development but just follow your child's lead. If he needs to nap, let him.

Quiet Time:

It is important for your child to have some quiet time in place of the nap that he has dropped. You may even notice that he occasionally falls asleep during quiet time. Create a cosy corner or space on the sofa where your child can look at books or play with some calm toys that are specifically reserved for quiet time. Television is generally quite stimulating but I found my eldest would settle nicely on the sofa with a gentle movie while his younger sister took a nap in her cot. Even at age four he regularly falls asleep with a movie for quiet time. I would not advise this as a nap but once the nap is dropped, it works well for the occasional snooze.

Remember – three and a half years is the average age to drop the nap completely so do not try to progress to dropping the nap too quickly because your child may become overtired and this may then affect his night-time sleep or cause early rising. Just because he manages a few days in a row without a nap, does not mean he is ready. Give it a few weeks and see what happens with bedtimes, night time and mornings too. If all stays on track, that's fine.

Nap transitions in day care:

Often day care providers advance children's naps too soon particularly when they are around age two and in the toddler's unit where some younger ones might need two hours or more while those closer to age three years, might only need to have an hour's nap. Again, at preschool age, many drop the nap completely before the child is really ready so be sure to communicate clearly with your day care provider as to how much sleep you would like them to accommodate for your child.

Sleep Nanny Note:

- Naps are very important. Especially for alert little ones.
- The total amount of daytime sleep and the way it is spread out really matters.
- A motion nap is better than no nap at all but the motion often maintains a lighter state of sleep.
- Nap quality and quantity are important.
- Nap training can be hard and slow but worth it.

Ditching The Dummy

Does your child use a dummy? How do you feel about it? How old is too old for a dummy?

So many parents say they won't let their child have one but then become a parent and realise the benefits of dummies for young babies. They are a source of great comfort and actually have been shown to reduce the risks of SIDS (sudden infant death syndrome). But at what stage does a dummy become a problem and how can you get rid of it?

There is really no harm in giving a baby a dummy. It supports their natural reflex to suckle and is comforting to them. As long as breastfeeding is established, breastfed newborns can have them too. Many babies come to rely on a dummy for sleep and many parents allow a dummy for sleep but not for any other time of day. This is good practice and if you have a rule like this stick to it. If you bend the rules for one reason one day, he will expect the rules can be bent anytime if he makes enough fuss.

Using a dummy for sleep can be very helpful but it can also become a hindrance. If a baby uses a dummy as a comfort to settle to sleep, that is fine. If a baby NEEDS a dummy to get back to sleep AND needs YOU to plug it back in – the dummy has become a sleep crutch and you need to address this.

Here are the rules:

Baby has a dummy to fall asleep and, once asleep, it drops out. Do not replace the dummy for him.

Encourage your baby to be in control of his dummy use – this will be age dependent but once he has the pincer grasp, he should find and replace his own dummy. You can encourage this by showing him where it is or temporarily putting it in his hand and then eventually just pointing at it so that he learns that he has to do it himself.

Some people put a number of dummies in the cot to make it easier for baby to find one.

If your baby is too young to replace his dummy himself, once it falls out, you leave it out. This sounds scary to parents because replacing it feels like the path of least resistance to get him back to sleep. That may be true right now but by ingraining this sleep crutch, you will be stuck doing the 'dummy run' all night for many, many months. Get this right now and it will pay off much sooner!

When should I get rid of the dummy?

This is a personal decision but most people do not enjoy seeing a toddler learning to talk with a dummy in her mouth. Even the parents who have an older toddler with a dummy usually do not like it but just do not know how to go about getting rid of it.

The benefits of a dummy for young babies are not so effective once they reach six to twelve months and the SIDS risks subside anyway.

If the dummy becomes a hindrance, it is time to say goodbye to it. It may be a hindrance with speech, with eating or with sleep. My own son's reliance on a dummy for sleep was the very thing that was causing him to wake in the night. When we took it away, he slept through the night on night one without it! It was more of a disturbance for him to lose the dummy in the night and want it back than it was to just deal with no longer having it. Sometimes there comes a point when it is no longer a sleep aid but a sleep hindrance.

How can I go about actually getting rid of the dummy completely?

There is no such thing as weaning a dummy. Children rarely give up the dummy of their own accord until aged five years or so, when school and peer pressure come into play. So it is up to you to take action if you want the dummy to go. The only way is 'cold turkey' and often the parents are more attached to the dummy than the child because of the parents' fear of the repercussions is far worse than the child's actual reaction.

If your child is old enough to understand a basic story, and even if they are not, because they will still pick up on a lot more than you realise – it can be a nice idea to tell a little story about why all the dummies have gone now and they won't be there any more.

Some examples:

- The fairies have to take them to all the new babies that are being born.
- Santa or the Easter bunny will swap them for gifts/eggs if you leave them out for them to take away.
- 'You're so clever that you don't need them any more so they have gone to the little babies who need them now.' (Avoid 'grown up' because not all children are happy about being grown up and want to still be your baby – which of course they are.)

You can be as creative as you like and use something your child can relate to. There is no need to frighten your child with any great dummy funeral or have the child throw them in the bin as that can be a bit dramatic and sad for them. Just make them all disappear and then tell the child calmly and reassuringly. It can be a nice gesture to have a gift or reward for your child when you break the news for being so brave about it.

It may take a few days for your child to adjust. Some accept the change faster than others and often the older they are the more difficult it is for them to 'kick the habit' but they all get there in probably less time than parents expect them to.

No going back: Once you make this move, you cannot go back. Not for any reason or excuse. If you do, your child will find it very hard to believe you mean it, next time you try. For you own sake, you must get shot of them all to remove all temptation of pulling one out in the heat of a challenging moment.

Be brave, do it today!

Sleep Nanny Note:

- Dummies serve little purpose past the age of six months.
- The most effective way to get rid of the dummy is to go 'cold turkey'.
- As children get older, dummies can affect teeth and speech.
- Parents often get as attached to the dummy as the baby or toddler.

Case Study: Amelie aged 7 months.

Amelie was very attached to her dummy for sleep but her parents found themselves having to go in and replace it for her several times through the night because she could not yet find it or put it back in by herself. Usually, replacing the dummy would be all Amelie needed and then everyone could go back to sleep but sometimes this would happen four to five times in an hour or Amelie would need more than just the dummy so her parents would pick her up and try to cuddle or rock her back to sleep – sometimes this worked and sometimes not so, as a last resort they would take her into their bed for the rest of the night.

We looked at the options for the dummy:

- Keep it in our plan and teach her how to take control of it herself. – This would be tricky because many babies are not able to grasp or make this complex move until around the age of nine months.
- Get rid of the dummy completely. – It bears little benefit past the age of six months and is likely to be increasing Amelie's disturbances in the night.

The parents were nervous about ditching the dummy. They feared this would mean Amelie would be awake and crying or screaming for hours on end in the night without this means of comfort. Having made this bold move myself in the past with my eldest, I knew exactly how they felt but I reassured them and explained that there was no easy time to do it and it only got harder the older they got so now was as good a time as any. They agreed that it was likely to be a good move and bravely they threw away all the dummies and gave Amelie a new bedtime teddy bear as a reward.

At first Amelie did look for the dummy when she woke, naturally, it was all she knew up until then. However after a few days of receiving comfort and reassurance from her parents while remaining in her cot, the dummy was forgotten. The parents' fears of having to spend long hours trying to resettle her in the night without having a dummy to give her and without taking her into their own bed, were quickly dashed because Amelie rapidly reduced her night waking and by night three she was sleeping through the night!

In this case, the dummy was actually the primary cause of the night waking and was hindering more than it was helping, even though it seemed to be the thing that most aided Amelie's sleep.

Night Weaning

Firstly you need to decide whether or not your baby still needs a feed in the night. I find it rare that a baby over eight months still needs a feed but it can happen. Many don't need a night feed from as young as three - four months so you need to know what your child actually needs, not wants for comfort, but actually needs through hunger. Usually your observations and instincts will tell you. If he is getting enough calories during the day and is in good health and weight, he may not need a night feed any more. Consult with your health visitor or doctor if you are unsure because it can be difficult to tell even a baby who is not hungry, might still take a large feed if it is offered. Imagine you woke up at 3 a.m. and somebody gave you a milkshake. You might not want it but you would probably be able to find room for it. If you decide that a night feed is no longer required but is something he still enjoys, here are some ways to wean it.

Cold Turkey - a simple and clear message, you close up shop on the milk after the bedtime feed and that is it until morning. If you choose this approach, mean it and don't second-guess yourself or give in when it gets tough. It can be hard work comforting them instead of feeding them when the feed is what they are used to, but it will be a quick solution if you stick to it.

Two-Step Drop - whether you're breastfeeding or bottle feeding, just give one feed per night for three nights. It's best to choose a consistent time for this feed so either make it, the first time she wakes after a set time like midnight, or the first time she wakes as long as it has been at least four hours since the last feed, or make it a dream feed that you do right before you go to bed without even waking her intentionally. Just make sure you only feed once at night and nothing more until at least 6 a.m. or upon starting your day. On the fourth night, don't feed at all. She has had three nights of adjusting to fewer calories through the night. If you're doing the Four-Step Fade-Out method and you do this night weaning method from the start, you can modify night four and do one extra night next to the cot to offer extra support and comfort if she wakes in the night – instead of giving a feed.

An important note on this method, if you are comforting your baby through a night waking and then it reaches that time when you decided it would be suitable to give the one feed, don't just give it right away, see your comforting through until she is back asleep and wait until the next waking to give the feed. Otherwise you'll give the message that you might soothe her for a bit and then resort to giving a feed anyway – not a message you want to convey!

Dream Feeding - This works really well with sleep training because you offer your baby a feed when she is asleep, rather than responding to a cry with a feed. You feel reassured that you know your baby has had enough calories and will not be hungry for the rest of the night which encourages you to be consistent with your soothing response to your baby's cries each and every time she wakes in the night.

Milk Reduction - If breastfeeding, this would mean gradually cutting down on the amount of time your baby is at each breast. You can cut back by five minutes each night until she is not bothered or if you get down to just five minutes, it might be a bit of a tease and better to stop altogether. Also, remember to unlatch her when she finishes eating heartily even if it is sooner than the allotted time and don't just let her comfort suckle and doze. If you are formula feeding you can decrease the amount in the bottle by a few ounces every few nights and when you get to two ounces, it's time to stop. Alternatively, you could dilute the formula with water making it gradually weaker each night until she is not even bothered about waking up for it. I find that some babies don't care what is in the bottle and just like to suckle so reducing the total amount works better.

Gradual Decrease - If you are not sure whether or not your baby still needs some calories in the night, you could follow the 'Milk Reduction' method above and once down to an amount that seems substantial enough, move to the Two-Step Drop' method but remain on one feed per night for a little longer if necessary. Doing it this way is more gradual and enables you to reduce rather than completely drop night feeding for the time being.

Sleep Nanny Note:

- Pay attention to whether your baby is hungry in the night or simply comfort suckling.
- Be sure your little one is getting enough calories during the day before night weaning.
- Choose a method that feels right for you and then stick with it.
- Always remember that feeding is more important than sleep.
- Babies can take a big feed in the night even when they are not really hungry.

Case Study: Jacob aged 5 months.

Jacob was still waking frequently in the night at five months and would feed almost every 2-3 hours after about 11 p.m. Jacob was a very healthy weight and size and was getting plenty of calories during the day and the large amount he was consuming in the night was actually making him digestively uncomfortable as well as soaking through his nappy most nights!

We did not want to simply stop all night feeds at once because there was a chance that Jacob could still be hungry in the night but we knew he did not need to feed as frequently through the night as he was. It was very clear that a lot of these feeds were for comfort so we needed to devise a new response to Jacob's cries and to comfort him in another way rather than always feed him.

We started out by offering a dream feed at 11 p.m. each night and the option of a second feed, if he woke after 3 a.m. and seemed hungry (which was very hard to tell). Our plan was to meet all other night wakings with a new response of comforting him within his cot by shh-ing him and stroking him intermittently for no more than 20 seconds and then sitting close by to continue shh-ing as needed.

On the first night, Jacob had the dream feed at 11 p.m. and then woke five times between midnight and 6 a.m. Each time he woke, his mum went in to comfort him and stayed with him until he went back to sleep as per our plan. It took 20-40 minutes most times but by 4 a.m. he seemed to have more willpower. After a second feed at 3.45 a.m. Jacob returned to sleep for a further hour and 20 minutes and this time it took an hour for him to resettle but he did it, which was so clever of him and well worth mum sticking it out because he really needed a bitter sleep.

After five nights of our plan, Jacob was accepting the dream feed and had only had a second feed on two nights. Mum had used other techniques to comfort him when he woke in the night and she stuck to it no matter how long it took each time. The longest it took Jacob to resettle in the first five nights was one hour and 42 minutes but on average he could resettle within 30 minutes.

As Jacob was getting better and better at resettling in the night, mum decided he did not really need a second feed and had only been using it for comfort. We agreed that we would try just the one dream feed and then no more feeding until morning which would also make for a much clearer message to Jacob because he would then get total consistency in the response he received when he woke and cried out in the night. If every night waking is met with the same response it is likely that it will take less and less time for a little one to resettle because they will stop holding out for the alternative outcome (such as a feed) that they might be hoping for.

Within two further nights (night seven), Jacob was doing fine on just one feed, had reduced his night waking down to just three wakings on average in the night and was resettling to sleep within 20 minutes each time; such an improvement in one week.

Whilst the nights were improving we still had some work to do on daytime naps. Jacob's naps had previously been quite irregular. Some days he would nap for a total of three to four hours while other days he would battle through the day on just two short 30 minute naps and be exhausted. We applied our night-time plan to naps and began working on one nap each day in his cot then increased to two naps in the cot by day five. The other naps were 'motion naps' so either took place in the pushchair or the car seat while on the go. This was better than no nap at all even if the quality of sleep is not likely to be so good.

We were aiming for Jacob to be getting three and a half to four hours of daytime sleep each day and we had to experiment a little to find his optimum windows for his naps. This took just over two weeks to settle into more of a rhythm and a further four weeks to really click into place. It is quite normal for naps to settle on track a little after night-time sleep improves but it is still important to fill up the 'sleep tank' during the day to avoid over tiredness which will then impact the night-time sleep.

By day 14, Jacob was going to bed at 7 p.m. and sleeping through to 6.00 a.m. with just one dream feed at 11 p.m. and at most, one night waking which he would resettle within five minutes and did not always need a parent to go to him either. He was taking three good naps every day, two of which would be in his cot and the third would often be out and about.

Self Settling

What does it mean to self settle and why is this the cornerstone to all sleep training? The ability to settle oneself to sleep is a learned skill. From birth a baby doesn't know how to do this and needs to be shown and taught in a way that is suitable for their age and development. Until a child can do this, he will rely on external help, like you, to do it for him. Once a baby learns and masters the skill of self settling, all the other pieces of sleep training come together quite nicely. Some babies learn to self settle much earlier than others and it often depends on the level of help they become used to after the early weeks.

If a baby is unable to settle to sleep without this help, he will require the help each and every time he wakes up in the night which might be after every sleep cycle or every few hours! Often, parents mistakenly think they have a hungry baby who needs to be fed every two hours all night long or they think they have a fussy baby who doesn't like sleep, when in actual fact, their baby just doesn't know how to get back to sleep and needs that help that he received at bedtime because it is the only way he knows how.

Teaching a baby how to self settle does not require leaving him alone to cry. Like any new task we face, we would all prefer to be guided and supported as we learn rather than left alone, feeling frustrated while we try to figure it out from scratch! Teaching your baby how to sleep independently can be achieved in a very gentle, kind and supportive manner with you responding to your child, reassuring and comforting him too. The change is not to take this support away but just to stop doing if FOR him.

Sleep Nanny Note:

- Self settling is a learned skill.
- You do not have to be cruel or leave a baby to cry in order to teach him to self settle.
- Self settling to sleep is a form of selfregulation and a vital life skill.

Consistency

Consistency is crucial. You may have heard before that consistency is key in sleep training but what does it really mean to be consistent and what happens if you are not? I want to share with you the difference it makes to your child when you are consistent, and the messages you send when you are not.

First, let's look at the dictionary definition of the word:

"1. Consistent behaviour or treatment: The quality of receiving a level of performance which does not vary greatly in quality over time."

It is important to be consistent in how you respond to your child in order to be fair to them. If they get inconsistent responses, they do not know where they stand and this can lead to frustration and misbehaving.

Example:
A parent will bring her baby into her bed but only around or after 5 a.m. when she is too deeply sleepy and too tired to try anything else to get the little one back to sleep. She feels it is the path of least resistance that will enable the whole family more sleep rather than battling with baby and waking everyone up – sound familiar?

This is a problem because babies cannot tell the time and do not understand when it is or is not okay to be taken into mum and dad's bed. All they understand is that is something they can 'get' if they cry so they will wake earlier and earlier and hold out longer for this result because they know it can happen.

So what should you do in this scenario? Follow my advice on early risers for your child's age and work out the most appropriate way to teach him to fall back to sleep. Yes it is tough work because we are most groggy around the 5 a.m. mark but it is a short-term pain for a long-term gain, I assure you – I've done it!

The same applies to boundaries which toddlers are particularly keen to test… If you allow one story at bedtime most nights but occasionally she asks for another one and you agree, you can bet your bottom dollar that she will ask for another and another next time. Then, when you say no and remind her that you only have one story at bedtime, she will be confused and might get angry or frustrated with your attempt to stick to this rule again.

This is called intermittent reinforcement – which basically means that on occasions, you bend the rules and thus reinforce your child's belief that the rules don't really stand.

Imagine a parent who decides to ditch the dummy and they explain to their toddler that there is no more dummy and battle through day one without it. Obviously this change is a little unsettling for a young child so they are likely to protest a bit but they will soon accept the change if you stick to your guns and keep moving forward. However, I have known parents do this and then hit a wall where they just cannot take the protesting any more, so they dig out a dummy they had stashed away and let the child have it. – Disaster! This child has just learned that if he makes enough fuss and noise about it, he will get it back. When this parent decides the dummy really has to go, this child is going to protest even harder and for longer. Either that or he will have the dummy until he goes to school! He also learns that you do not mean what you say which can lead to further behaviour struggles later on if this pattern continues.

I have caught myself saying 'no' to something to my children and then reconsidering it thinking 'actually, it's no big deal, I could have said yes to that' but I remind myself it is too late now and I must stick to my word. If I changed my mind now, my children would learn that after ten times 'no' you get a 'yes' so just keep nagging, whinging or crying. I like to call this the no, no, no, no, no, no, oh alright then, mistake.

So we have explored what consistency is and the effects of intermittent reinforcement and you can apply this to every area of parenting but it is so important when you start to work on sleep training. Be sure about what your plan is so that you can be consistent with it and don't start something you cannot follow through with.

Sleep Nanny Note:

- Consistency is key in most areas of parenting as it sends clear rather than conflicting messages.
- Being inconsistent will confuse a child and encourage him to hold out for the result he knows he sometimes gets.
- It is better to not start something unless you can be consistent in seeing it through.

Average Sleep Needs By Age

Understanding how much sleep your little one needs for their age is really powerful information. It will help you to identify when they are most ready to take naps, how long they need to sleep during the day and at night, and generally make it easier to structure your day while accommodating your child's sleep needs. Look at my chart of average sleep needs to find out what is ideal for your own child.

Age	Total Sleep	Total Night-time Sleep	Total Daytime Sleep	Number of naps	Wakeful Window	Average per nap length
0-5 months	15 1/2 hrs	8 1/2 hrs	Varies	4-5 /day	45mins-2hrs	Varies
6-8 months	14 1/2 hrs	11 hrs	3 1/4 hrs	3 /day	1.5-3 hrs	1-1.5hrs
9-11 months	14 hrs	11 hrs	3 hrs	2 / day	2-4 hrs	1.5hrs
12-18 months	13 1/2 hrs	11 1/4 hrs	2 1/2 hrs	1-2 /day	4-6 hrs	1-2.5hrs
2 years	13 hrs	11 hrs	1 1/2 - 2 hrs	1 /day	5-6 hrs	1.5-2 hrs
3 years	12 hrs	10 1/2 hrs	30 mins - 1 1/2 hrs	1 nap/QT	6+ hrs	30m-1.5 hrs
4 years	11 1/2 hrs	11 1/2 hrs	Quiet Time	1 nap/QT	-	varies
5 years	11 hrs	11 hrs	Quiet Time	QT	-	-
6 years	10 3/4 hrs	10 3/4 hrs	Quiet Time	QT	-	-

Note down how much total night-time sleep your child needs, how much total daytime sleep and in how many naps. Also take a note of how long her wakeful window is likely to last before she needs another sleep. Based on what time your child usually wakes up, and if this is all over the place, go with the time you are aiming for as wake-up time. So based on that time and how long the wakeful window is, what time should the first nap occur? Make a note of this. Then, to work out how long this nap should last, look at how much total daytime sleep is needed and in how many naps, so, if it is three hours over two naps, you might want to aim for nap one lasting between one hour and one and a half hours then repeat the wakeful duration in order to see when roughly the next nap should occur and again, you can work out roughly how long you are aiming for this nap to last.

Here is an example for a 10-month-old baby:
- Baby wakes up at 6.30 a.m. and has a wakeful window of three hours.
- Ready for nap one by 9.30 a.m. and this nap to last 90 minutes.
- Awake for three hours.
- Ready for nap two by 14:00 and this nap to last 90 minutes.
- Awake for three and a half hours.
- Bedtime at 7 p.m.
- Total daytime sleep = three hours over two naps.
- Total night-time sleep = 11.5 hours.

Remember, this is what you are aiming for, it won't be that simple to start with because, no doubt your child won't nap for as long as he is supposed to and will throw off your ideal schedule. Don't panic, as he refines his sleep skills from your night-time plan, he will start to stretch out the naps to the more appropriate lengths. It will take time, but this will help you to map out what you are aiming for.

Sleep And Wakeful Windows

Knowing your child's optimum sleep windows can make a huge difference to how easily they settle to sleep and how long they stay asleep. What if all you needed to was to find those windows? How much smoother could naps and bedtime be for everyone?

So what is a sleep window exactly?

Depending on your baby or child's age, there will be an average amount of time she can manage to be awake in any one stretch. For example, a six-month-old will manage around 1.5-2hrs awake before needing another sleep. When you attempt to put your baby down for a sleep too soon, she may protest as she is not ready yet. If you miss the window and try after the window closes, she will protest because she is now overtired and the brain has released the hormone, cortisol to keep her awake!

If there is no sign of a nap coming, bright lights, noise, TV and lots of stimulation, the brain thinks we need to wake up and releases cortisol, which is like adrenaline. This is why your child may *seem* wide awake or wired when they are actually overtired.

So how do we catch the sleep windows?

For many alert little ones, it can be hard to spot their sleepy cues as they are very good at hiding them. Knowing roughly when to expect them to be tired can make it easier to spot the optimum window but sometimes they still show no signs so you just have to go with the timing and try. With a bit of trial and error, you can soon work out when your baby's optimum sleep windows are.

When you find the sleep windows it is like a surfer catching a wave – get it just right and you will ride it all the way to the shore.

How can you do this with your little one?

- Use my table on page 75 to find the average sleep amount needed for your child's age (night and naps).
- Use the table to also find out the average wakeful window for your child's age.
- Accommodate your child's sleep schedule as best as you can so that he is not awake for too long in one stretch and is getting enough total sleep.

You will be amazed at the difference in your baby's ability to settle more easily and sleep for longer when you find the right spot!

How To Keep Your Child In Their Own Bed All Night

Most babies and young children will prefer to be near you rather than in a room by themselves but it is healthy for us to all have our own space and for a child to feel safe and happy in their own room. Also, when you have a large family, it is not possible for you all to be in one room or one bed, even if it is a super king-sized! This chapter is for people who are not looking to co-sleep and want to actively encourage their child to stay in their own bed/room all night.

When parents tell me their child won't stay in his own bed, my first questions are, how old is he and is he in a cot or a bed? There is a big difference between a child who is independently choosing to get up and out of his bed to a baby or child in a cot who is holding out for you to make the decision to take him out and bring him in with you.

Firstly let's look at the toddlers in a bed. They do not gain the cognitive ability to understand the concept of 'staying in bed' until they are at least two and a half years old. If your toddler is below this age it may be a bigger challenge to train her to stay in bed, depending on her temperament. If your child is above this age, you can try the following techniques:

1. Rapid Return (for toddlers and young children in beds)
This is an approach used for a child who is repeatedly getting out of bed. You take them by the hand and lead them quickly and quietly back to bed without engaging in any kind of conversation, minimal eye contact and no cuddles after the initial 'night-night' at bedtime. The idea is that they begin to find no reason to get up again because

they are not getting the response from you that they are looking for. If the child is old enough, you can also tell him that you will only tuck him in once and if he gets up again, he will have to do it himself. This approach is really effective when used alongside a reward system or a sticker chart.

Key points:
- You must remain consistent in your actions for each return and not get drawn into a conversation or negotiation – toddlers are good at that!
- You should have a conversation about what you expect from your child before you leave them at bedtime so there is no need to discuss it again when they get up.
- Requires patience.

2. Gating the Door

Make the bedroom completely safe and put a stair gate across the door so that your child's bedroom becomes like a large-scale cot. After you put your child to bed, close the door and then sit in the hallway the other side of the gate. Each time your child gets up and comes to the gate, whisper to him to get back into bed or simply just point to his bed and gesture. Do not interact or engage in any kind of conversation or negotiation. If he asks to be tucked in, you can tell him that you will tuck him in once and if he gets up again, he will have to tuck himself back in. Stick to your guns!

It can be hard to keep your cool but do try not to show your frustration. Be patient but firm and be totally boring to your child so that he has nothing to get up for. He needs his sleep and you are doing the best thing for him by teaching him to settle in his own bed.

3. Sleep Manners Reward System

You can create a chart with four or five 'sleep manners' in a column on the left-hand side and the days of the week across the top. There will be a space every morning to place a sticker for each sleep manner that your child achieved that night.

It is a good idea to make one of the sleep manners fairly easy to achieve so he can experience a sense of pride right away. My suggested sleep manners are:

- Co-operated at bedtime
- Put myself to sleep quietly at bedtime
- Put myself back to sleep in the night without any help from Mummy or Daddy
- Stayed quietly in bed until getting up time (perhaps to be signalled by a day/night clock)

At bedtime, go through the chart with your child and make sure he knows what each of the sleep manners are. You can even ask him and have him tell you. Use positive and encouraging language around this such as 'I know you can do it' and 'it will be great to see four stickers on the chart in the morning'. Avoid any negative talk of disappointment or consequences. Your child should run through the chart first thing in the morning with you and receive one sticker for each sleep manner achieved. You may wish to reward him for getting all four in the morning or for completing the whole week once he gets the hang of it. If you do use a reward or prize, make it something your child is really into and that means something to him. The stronger the incentive, the more likely he is to accomplish this. It is amazing what they can do when they really want to! It also helps if the prize is visible to your child so if you can put it on a high shelf somewhere he can see it but not touch it, even show him and then put it away, and tell him it will be his when he completes all four stickers in the morning or the whole week with no gaps will work well once he gets the hang of it.

Don't be afraid to let him feel a bit of disappointment on the occasions when he misses one. Make it clear that he did not achieve that sticker, suggest he can do it tonight and then move on without dwelling on it. It is this little feeling of pain that will drive him to accomplish the task.

This method is one worth sticking with as it can take a while for a child to get into it. It is also one you can bring back anytime they have a phase of testing you again.

Sleep Manners	Mon	Tue	Wed	Thu	Fri	Sat	Sun
Co-operated at bedtime							
Stayed in bed and quietly put self to sleep							
Put self back to sleep in the night without help from Mummy/Daddy							
Stayed in bed quietly until wake-up time							

In a cot but won't stay there all night?

If your little one is still in a cot (and not climbing out) but always ends up in your bed with you at some stage of the night, this is totally in your hands. Find the right soothing approach to suit her temperament and work on resettling her in her own cot. That might mean sitting with her until she goes back to sleep and perhaps adopting the Four-Step Fade Out or it could be that Regulated Responding would be better suited (see Selecting Your Gentle Sleep Training Approach on page 35). The important thing is that you choose how you will respond to all night waking and then stick to it.

It might seem like the fastest way to get everyone back to sleep is to just bring your baby into your bed with you. In some cases it is and in other cases no-one gets any more sleep anyway. But long term, this is not going to serve you so it may mean undergoing a short-term pain for a long-term gain.

I often hear parents say of their baby in a cot, 'she just _seems_ to end up in our bed every night'. If you are the one taking her there, she doesn't 'seem' to end up there, you are choosing to bring her there.

Do you have an escape artist?

Some toddlers seem to be able to break out of anything! I once spoke to a mother who told me her little boy could open his car seat straps and get out of his seat at just 13 months. Terrifying when she was on the motorway! Fortunately I have only heard of this once and I would be questioning the security of that car seat but it is quite common for toddlers to start climbing out of the cot or over a stair gate. So what should you do?

First of all look at ways to keep her in the cot rather than rushing to a toddler bed too soon because that could just open a whole new can of worms for you. Have you tried using a sleep sack? It is very hard to get out when the legs are zipped up in one of these. Or, there are some pyjamas on the market now that have a very low crutch specifically designed to prevent cot climbers from getting their legs up to the top of the cot side. Is the cot large enough? Travel cots or pack 'n' plays are much easier for a toddler to climb out of than a standard sized cot with the mattress on the lowest setting. Also, perhaps see if you can swap your cot with someone and try a different style. My own daughter found she could climb out of the cot at grandma's house but not at home. The cots were the same size but for some reason she didn't feel comfortable seeing through her attempt to climb out of the one at home. It might be worth cushioning any falls with a soft landing pad while you monitor your child's climbing progress.

If you have covered all these bases and your little one still continues to climb out or it gets to the point of being unsafe to keep her in a cot, then you will probably have to look at transitioning to a bed a bit on the early side but prepare to be patient as you may experience some difficulty keeping her in there because the approaches detailed earlier in this chapter may be too difficult for her to understand at this age.

Sleep Nanny Note:

- Be clear about where you want your child to sleep and stick to it.
- Use age appropriate techniques to keep your child in her own bed all night.
- Ensure your climbing or wandering child is safe.
- Children under the age of two and a half do not have the cognitive ability to understand the concept of staying in bed.
- Only bed share if you are happy to do this at any hour.

How To Get Yourself Back To Sleep After A Disturbance

It is one thing learning about how to resettle your child but what about us parents? Have you ever been disturbed by your little one who quickly went back to sleep, leaving you lying there wide awake for the next hour or more? One night, when this happened to me, I started to think about how I could help parents with this problem. As I lay there, I remembered some of the techniques I had learned when I practised hypnobirthing with my first baby. These techniques put me into a complete state of relaxation and calm and often I would nod off to sleep while practicing them. To test it out, I began to use the sleep breathing technique and in no time I was back to sleep. I woke up that morning feeling delighted that I had found a way to help parents get back to sleep in the night!

When we are disturbed in the night it can set the mind racing with thoughts and concerns that cause us tension, such as, 'is he going to wake up again?' or 'should I have done that?' or even just the frustration of being awake and wanting to go back to sleep. This tension then makes it much more difficult for us to relax and go back to sleep. So let's have a look at how to use these techniques which are taken from 'Hypnobirthing' by Marie Mongan.

Facial Relaxation

Marie Mongan explains that facial relaxation will set the tone for the rest of your body. Here is her description of how to achieve this:

'*...Let your eyelids slowly close. Don't try to force them shut, just let them gently meet. Place your awareness on the muscles in and around your eyes. As you feel a natural drooping of the eye muscles, sense relaxation spreading from your forehead, down across your eyelids, over your cheekbones and around your jaws. Let your lower jaw recede as your teeth part. Relax your tongue. Your eyelids will feel heavier as your cheeks and your jaw go limp. Bring the relaxation within your eyes to a level where it will seem as though your eyelids just refuse to work. Place the tip of your tongue at your palate where your upper teeth and palate meet, bringing about a sense of peace and well-being as you connect with your energy body. Feel your head making a dent into the pillow. As you practice this technique, you will feel your neck, your shoulders and your elbows droop. Picture your shoulders opening outward and sinking down into the frame of your body as you go deeply into relaxation...*'

Sleep Breathing

Sleep breathing helps to relax the body and the mind by quietening all that inner 'chatter'. This breathing is done with the mouth closed or partially open through facial relaxation and all breathing is through the nose.

Slowly draw in a breath from your stomach to the count of four (in-2-3-4), as you breathe in, feel your stomach rise and draw the breath up into the back of your throat. Pause, and then exhale very slowly through your nose, to the count of eight (out-2-3-4-5-6-7-8). As you breathe out, direct the energy of the breath down and inward, toward the back of your throat. Relax and let go, feeling yourself sink into your pillow and bed.

With practise, you will master this technique and not need to count and you will find it will take you into relaxation very quickly once you get the hang of it. I recommend trying this out during the day when you get a quiet 10 minutes. It can also be a great way to unwind and release some tension while your baby takes a nap.

Sleep Nanny Note:

- Try to unwind and have some relaxing time before you go to bed.
- If you have a busy mind, keep a notepad by your bed and jot down any thoughts that are keeping you from going back to sleep.
- Use the sleep breathing technique.

Sleep Regressions, Developmental Leaps And Fussy Phases

What is a sleep regression? If your baby goes from sleeping through the night to suddenly waking several times or can no longer fall asleep or stay asleep, fights naps and is expressing the three C's: Crying, Clingy and Cranky, you have ruled out any illness or teething and it has lasted more than a few days like a growth spurt... this may well be a sleep regression.

When do they occur? The most common sleep regressions occur around 4-6 months, 8-10 months and 11-13 months. Typically around the times a baby learns to roll, to crawl and to walk. At these stages, your baby goes through tremendous cognitive development and while learning the new skill, she will practise it again and again, even in her head, until she masters it.

Why does this affect sleep? Imagine how you feel when you are really excited about something or really nervous about a big event. You cannot turn off your thoughts which often keep you awake at night. During these phases for a baby, the brain is in overdrive and similarly, they cannot shut it off and find it really hard to get to sleep. This results in a tired, cranky baby the next day.

What can you do? Firstly, remember that this will not last forever and, if you have already got a well-trained little sleeper, things will get back on track quite quickly as long as you stay consistent. Remember to stick to your routine, especially at bedtime and don't be afraid to offer a little more reassurance than usual. Respond to your baby's cries and comfort her but avoid reverting back to any old sleep crutches that you have done away with. Also, encourage her with her new skill to help her to master it with plenty of practise during the day.

Sometimes a sleep regression will highlight the lack of a sleep skill such as your baby being unable to settle himself to sleep and relying on you to do it for him. In this instance, devise your plan to help him learn this skill and begin to implement your plan as soon as possible. This skill will help him pass through a sleep regression faster but it may take until the regression has passed before he shows you that he can do it.

A baby's sleep may also take a regression as a result of a change in an area such as: routine, health, travel, physical development, mental development or environment. It is not possible to pinpoint when to expect these because it depends on so many variables. However, you can be aware of any changes that might disrupt your baby's sleep and offer reassurance and comfort through this phase; are they teething, just learned to walk, have you changed the routine?

The Wonder Weeks by Hetty van de Rijt and Frans Plooij defines the 10 predictable weeks in a baby's mental development during the first 20 months. These are based on lots of research and neurological studies that show significant changes in a baby's brain at, more or less, the same time for every child.

A developmental leap is usually preceded by a fussy phase and not knowing when to expect these can leave parents confused, confidence knocked and a bewildered baby. For physical development, these will happen at various ages because one child may start to walk at 10 months while another may not walk until 18 months. However, studies show that you can predict the mental developmental leaps to within a week or two! (*The Wonder Weeks.*)

According to *The Wonder Weeks*, you can expect a fussy phase at weeks; 5, 8, 12, 15, 23, 34, 42, 51, 60 and 71. These are based on changes in the nervous system from conception but the weeks listed have been calculated from date of birth. Therefore, you should adjust these for your baby if he was premature or very late. The fussy phase can occur a week either side of these and may last anything from a few days to six weeks.

Whilst this is a useful guide, I don't like to get hung up on exact times to expect these phases. You could experience a fussy phase due to mental development followed by a fussy phase due to physical development and then a fussy phase caused by a disruption to the routine or due to ill health. It might feel like they come along one after the other and life seems to be one big fussy phase!

If you blame everything on a developmental leap, wonder week, or growth spurt, your child will never truly learn the sleep skills he really longs for. Sure, be aware of these phases and help your child through them but do not expect miracles on the other side if your baby was already lacking in the ability to sleep independently. On the flip side, if you have a skilled little sleeper, don't let these phases faze you (for want of a better phrase!), things will be back to normal in no time.

Sleep Nanny Note:

- Babies and young children with excellent sleep skills and self settling ability will be less thrown off track by developmental leaps.
- Knowing roughly when to expect a fussy phase can help you to make sense of it.
- Maintain routine and consistency through these phases as much as possible.

Nightmares, Night Terrors or Something Else?

The term 'night terrors' or sleep terrors can be thrown around a bit too easily when often it is actually a nightmare, a bad dream or a confusional arousal that your child is having. I have many parents ask me about night terrors but true night terrors are rarely seen in a child under the age of six years. They are more likely to occur in the preadolescent and adolescent years. So what is happening when your child has an upset waking in the night? Let's take a look at these different occurrences so that you can identify them properly.

Confusional events, known as parasomnias, include night terrors, sleepwalking, sleep talking and confusional arousals. These occur when the awake and sleep systems are trying to function simultaneously, like a battle between the waking system trying to activate and the sleep system not giving in to it. What we see when this happens is a child who demonstrates signs of being awake and of being asleep, at the same time.

We looked at baby sleep cycles on page 16 and how young children transition through non-REM and REM sleep. There are four stages of NREM sleep before REM sleep occurs. These four stages are:

Stage one: Transitioning from awake to asleep

Stage two: Light sleep

Stage three: Sleep deepens

Stage four: Deepest sleep takes place

Confusional events always take place during a partial waking from NREM sleep, before the transition to REM sleep and usually between one to four hours after falling asleep (often within the first two hours). So it is likely to be during the first or second sleep cycle of the night. They are quite common and, up to the age of five or six years, these confusional events are considered to be developmental because they reflect the maturing sleep system in a child.

You may notice some calm sleepwalking, sleep talking, or even getting up and seeming irritated but disorientated. These can all occur to different extents of calm or upset.

Confusional arousals are very often mistaken for night terrors.

These are some symptoms of a child having a confusional arousal:
- Thrashing his body
- Saying 'no, no, no' or 'get off' or 'go away' or similar
- Lashing out
- Crying out
- Upset
- Disorientated/Confused
- Cross/Angry
- Appears to be awake – eyes are open
- Looks right through you or doesn't recognise you
- Can be further irritated by your attempts to comfort him and may push you away
- Unlikely to respond to your questions
- Can seem frantic but not terrified

When children say alarming things such as 'no, no!' or 'stop it' during a confusional arousal this is nothing to worry about. It is coming from automatic vocal triggers in low areas of the brain and not from any areas that control waking or unconscious thoughts or anxieties.

Several demonstrations of confused arousal can occur in succession separated by just a few minutes of sleep before a calm and sustained sleep returns.

What should you do?

Don't try to wake your child as this is more likely to make things worse than better. Monitor him to make sure he is not going to hurt himself during the episode. If you feel you need to be with him, sit by his side and offer reassuring, calm whispers but be prepared to be shouted at or ignored as you may just become part of the confusion. He might talk nonsense to you but is unlikely to find any comfort in anything you say to him. All you can really do is wait for the episode to pass.

If they are up and out of bed, you can tell him or gently guide him back to bed and perhaps remain in the room quietly until the episode passes and he goes back to sleep.

Nightmares:

A nightmare is a very scary dream that wakes you up and leaves you feeling frightened. This begins as a normal dream but towards the end it turns scary. These, like all dreams, occur during REM sleep when the brain is more active and they are often forgotten. They are only remembered if there was a brief waking at the end of the dream or nightmare.

How can you help?

Younger children cannot distinguish a dream from reality until they are at least two years old so trying to reassure an under two-year-old with words like 'it was just a dream' is not going to help. Instead, you should offer comfort and reassurance by holding and hugging and soothing to calm your child down.

From the age of two years upwards reassuring words will help and listening to what they have to say if they want to tell you about it, will also offer comfort and compassion.

At around three - four years old you can remind your chid that it was just a dream and she will be able to understand this concept but still listen and empathise rather than dismiss it.

At any age, your child might take comfort from having a night light on so she can see around the room or having the bedroom door left open somewhat to feel more connected with the rest of the house and you. Your child will have woken up feeling genuinely scared so it is important to offer comfort and security and not to be too strict.

Confusional events are often linked to over tiredness. Perhaps from a late night or just a lack of sleep in the sleep tank that has built up. A few early nights or getting enough nap time could significantly reduce the chances of these occurring.

Monsters & 'Scaries':

It is very common among preschoolers to talk about monsters or other scary creatures hiding in their rooms. I am not a big fan of checking under the bed and in the cupboard to prove to your child there is nothing there, or the 'monster-away' sprays to repel any potential scary visitors. These just reinforce to your child the possibility of these things existing. Instead, I prefer to explain that they are not real and just pretend. Show your child that there is nothing under the bed or in the wardrobe if it makes them feel better but do this from a place of 'you see, I told you they are not real and there is nothing here' rather than you 'checking' for them. If you like the idea of a spray, instead of a monster-away spray, how about a good-dreams spray? Always focus on the positive. Most importantly and the most simple way to help a child who is worried about 'scaries' is to reinforce their sense of security, remind her that you are in charge and will always keep her safe in this safe place. Mention the other family members in the household who are there and remind her that you are all safe together and no-one else is there.

If nightmares occur several times per month or more frequently, perhaps you could spend some time during the day addressing what it is that is troubling her. Big changes such as moving house or starting school can bring about some insecurity. With a younger one, perhaps the fear is being alone so you could try some games like peek-a-boo to demonstrate that you are always nearby and will always return.

Sleep Nanny Note:

- Confusional arousals are quite common in young children aged three to eight years.
- It is unlikely your child will remember the event of a parasomnia in the morning.
- You can comfort a child waking from a nightmare but there is little you can do for a child experiencing a parasomnia such as a confusional arousal or night terror, other than keep him safe from physical harm.
- Over tiredness is a large contributor to these events.

Teething and Sleep

Teething alone is not a cause of sleep difficulties but it can contribute to disturbed nights much like any bodily pain or discomfort. One thing worth knowing is that when we suck, we draw blood to our gums which can increase the pain of teething so a dummy, bottle feeding or breastfeeding might add to the discomfort during this time. Biting down on something, like a teether for example, releases pressure from the gums which, in turn, eases the pain of teething.

Some children reject the dummy when they are teething while others want it more because they are using it to bite on. Watch your child to see what he instinctively does to soothe his gums and don't make any adjustments to sleep training during this phase until the worst has passed. At the same time, avoid bringing back any old sleep crutches or forms of comfort that you have moved past. Rather than go backwards, just 'stand still' in the sleep training process for a few days.

Of course there are medical forms of relief for teething pain but you should consult your doctor or pharmacist about choosing these and make sure they are age appropriate.

Siblings and Sleep

Whether you have twins or young siblings, it can be a challenge to teach one how to sleep if the other needs your attention or if one disturbs the other.

This can be particularly challenging if you are sleep training one, let alone two children at the same time! It can be made a lot easier with a two parents to two children ratio but that is not always possible, so what can you do?

Here are some tips to handling siblings and sleep with one pair of hands...

- Try to do their bedtime routine simultaneously.
- Give a preschool age or older child a book or a jigsaw to do quietly in his room while you put the younger one to bed.
- Read a bedtime story to the children together in one of their rooms, then take the youngest to bed and tell the older that you will be in to tuck them in shortly.
- Going to start sleep training? If you are on your own at sleep times, you will need a sleep training plan that is achievable and enables you to tend to the siblings as well as the child you are sleep training.
- If one child is more of a battle to settle at bedtime, settle the easier child first and praise his good behaviour. Then take your time with the more challenging child.
- Try not to bow down to every whim of a stalling toddler just because you fear she will disturb her sibling. It is amazing what they can sleep through. If old enough, you can always promise the sibling an extra goodnight kiss if they stay quietly

in bed until the challenging child has settled.

- If you have twins or singletons sharing a room and one just disturbs the other every time they try to settle, consider separating them temporarily (this may mean one in your room) until they are more skilled at settling to sleep.
- Don't feel you have to rush in to 'rescue' your baby at the slightest sound she makes. She may well fall back to sleep by herself and it is unlikely she will wake a sibling in deep sleep anyway.
- If one child naps but another doesn't, occupy the older child while you settle the younger napper and then reward the older child with some one-to-one attention while the little one naps.
- My own children are pretty close in age and are in rooms right next to each other. If Daddy is working late, I often do bedtime by myself and you will find you just get into a natural groove or flow that works for your family.

Parenting and Sleep

Do you consider yourself a strict parent or a soft touch? Or have you found a balance somewhere in the middle? It really doesn't matter where you sit on this scale as long as you have one key ingredient at all times… you guessed it, CONSISTENCY. Once you have a clear plan, which will be one you are comfortable with, you absolutely must stick to it, to the letter. Changing direction, giving in once you have said no, or giving more help to sleep than your plan allows, will all sabotage your attempts and elongate the process a great deal.

You need to have patience with sleep training. Your baby needs you to show him what is expected of him and support him while he learns. If you start something, you must see it through otherwise you may not be taken seriously next time. For example, I can think of many occasions when I have said no to something my son has asked for at bedtime. 20 minutes into a mega tantrum, I'll ask myself 'why didn't I just let him have it in the first place? Is it really that big a deal?' The problem is I have said no now and I cannot go back on this. Even though I know that if I just gave in we could all get to sleep a lot sooner – there's no turning back. No negotiating a compromise or meeting him halfway; time to ride out the storm and see it through. If I gave in, he would learn that he calls the shots and that he will do things his way and this will carry across his behaviour generally. So when he next asks for that thing at bedtime and I say no, he will create an even bigger storm and for longer because he learned last time that this does work eventually. Or, if I said yes this time, he would just add another request and another request to see how much control he has gained –they are clever little monkeys. The parent must stay in charge of the situation.

Implementation

If you are going to sleep train your child it is important to take a look at your parenting style and make sure this works in harmony with your sleep plan.

Ask yourself a few tough questions and answer with total honesty:
- Am I trying one technique such as controlled crying, in the evening and early part of the night but then bringing my child into my bed after 3 a.m.?
- Have I stopped night feeds but sometimes give a feed when I am desperate to go back to sleep at 4.30 a.m.?
- Do I sit by my baby's cot soothing her back to sleep and then give up after 30 minutes and just take her out of the cot and rock her to sleep in my arms?
- Do I sometimes leave my child to cry a bit and other times go in and pick him up?

If you have answered yes to any of these, you are displaying intermittent reinforcement, in other words, you are confusing your child. He cannot understand why things are 'sometimes' okay and other times not okay. He cannot tell the time so doesn't know when he is allowed to come into your bed and when he is not allowed. If sometimes you feed him, he will expect this result any time he chooses.

It's time to get very clear and very consistent.

Troubleshooting – The Baby Sleep Blueprint™

When you feel stuck or find yourself scratching your head over something that you just can't find the answer to, my Baby Sleep Blueprint™ below, will help to guide you. Always start with bedtime and this route map will guide you to your solutions.

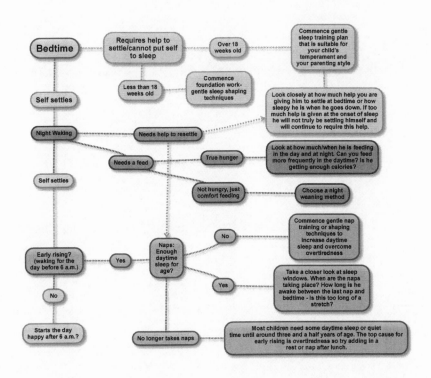

Travel Tips

A lot of parents worry about how their child's sleep will be affected when they travel but if your child sleeps well at home, he will be likely to sleep well on holiday or staying with family. If you have recently gone through a sleep coaching process with your child, it is advisable to have three weeks in your new routine at home after sleep coaching is complete, before travelling. This gives your child the chance to get fully adjusted to his new routine and well practised at his new skills before expecting him to manage these in a new environment.

When you travel, your child may slip back and show a few old sleep traits but try not to undo any of your hard work, for example by going back to whatever sleep crutch you have just eliminated or by feeding in the night when you had weaned him from night feeds. You may want to do a bit more soothing and comforting than you do at home but find a way to soothe your child that does not bring back the problem you began with. If you let your child do something on holiday (for example, sleep in your bed), he will be likely to want the same treatment when you get back home. If your toddler does sneak into your bed a few times and you are happy with this, just make sure he knows it is only okay in your holiday home as a special holiday treat, that way he won't expect the same treatment at home.

What to Take:
Take everything you need to make your child's sleep environment as similar to home as possible. Make sure you have the teddy or comfort blanket, night light, wake-up clock, and even your child's own pillow and blankets if you have room to pack them – unwashed so that they have the familiar smell from home. You'll need their favourite bedtime

stories and bath toys if possible. You want your child to have as much familiarity as possible, especially around the bedtime routine. It is also a great idea to take your baby monitor with you so that you feel assured that he is settled and you can perhaps relax on the veranda?

A sleep shade for your pushchair is great for blocking out the sun at nap time and acts as a great mosquito net too! You can also take a travel blackout blind if you think sunlight might be an issue in the bedroom.

Make sure the accommodation can provide you with a suitable cot or bed for your child. Not all countries have the same safety standards as we do so make sure you check over any cot provided. I would also suggest taking some antibacterial wipes for the cot sides and mattress.

Where to Sleep:

If you can separate your sleep space from that of your baby that would be ideal so that she does not wake up and see you straight away and want to play. With apartments you often get a separate bedroom or two and in hotels, interconnecting rooms are great and some family hotels even have a kids' room within the hotel room. If you are all in one room, try to be creative and make some sort of division between your bed and the baby's sleep space. I have even heard of mums hanging a sheet up to create a partition! Ideally you want to have your child sleep in the same place for the duration of the holiday.

Evenings:

If you are on holiday you are not likely to want to sit in your hotel room from 7 p.m. every night while your child is tucked up in bed. While it is ideal for your child to be in the room where they are going to spend the night, it is not a big problem to be flexible for a short time while you are away but try to make your 'holiday routine' a consistent one so that your child knows what to expect in this environment. So here are some suggestions that will depend on your child's age...

Young babies are very portable and if you take your lie-flat pram, you could do the bedtime routine and put baby down in the pram. Once she is settled to sleep you will find you can wheel her into a restaurant and possibly even enjoy some entertainment without her being disturbed. It is advisable to stick to the quieter areas if possible and not park her right next to a speaker! But you will find she will sleep through a fair amount of noise. The older they get the less likely this will work and if you find your baby does not stay asleep like this and is frequently disturbed, you may need to make this time short and get her back to the room in the quiet and look at some of the other suggestions below.

If your baby is too big for a pram but you have a reclining pushchair, you can do your bedtime routine and get your child into pyjamas and then settle them to sleep in the pushchair. Later you should be able to transfer your sleepy child, with little fuss, into the cot or bed as long as you minimise the interaction with them at this time.

If you have no luck with taking a sleeping child out in a pram or pushchair and you feel he really needs to be in the room, you may choose to take turns with a partner to stay in the room and read or if you have a balcony and weather permits, you can enjoy your evening on there with your children just inside.

Time Zones:

Travelling into a different time zone need not be as big a deal as you might think. I am not a big fan of the gradual method, adjusting your child's schedule in gradual increments – if you only have a week away or less, you do not have time for this. Also, the time you spend travelling is likely to throw your child's schedule right off, meaning you have a reasonable 'blank canvas' to work with when you get there. The fact that the sun is up or down will also signal to your child what time of day it is and begin adjusting their circadian rhythms (internal body clock) so you might as well move to local time as soon as you arrive and vice versa when you go home. As long as you have your consistent 'holiday routine', you will see your child very quickly adjust. Just keep an eye on your child's sleepy cues and allow your child any extra naps needed after travel or bring bedtime forward a little if they need to catch up.

Enjoy:

Whilst it is not easy travelling with small children, it can still be a lovely way to get a break away and enjoy some quality family time, so enjoy it. Yes, routines and consistency are important but not to the extent that it ruins your holiday. Your child will soon get back to normal when you return home and if you do need to do a little bit of retraining in the sleep department, it will be much quicker and easier than first time round.

Daylight Savings – Clock Changes

Spring Forward:

Are you dreading the clocks going forward one hour? Or are you excited at the idea of your child's wake-up time shifting from 6.30 a.m. to 7.30 a.m.? Every time we change our clocks, parents worry about the affects it might have on their children and wonder how best to deal with the change. You have three options:

- 'Cold turkey' just shift to the new time straight off. Many children adapt well this way and it has no effect on them. If bedtime is normally 7 p.m., just put your child down at 6 p.m. on Saturday night. Great for easy-going and flexible temperaments.
- Gradually move your child's bedtime earlier in 15 minute increments on the four nights leading up to the clock change. E.G. if normal bedtime is 7 p.m., put him down at 6.45 on Wednesday night, 6.30 on Thursday night, 6.15 on Friday night and 6 p.m. on Saturday night. This works well for those more sensitive temperaments.
- Split the difference and put your child to bed 30 minutes earlier. So, based on a normal 7 p.m. bedtime, put her down at 6.30 p.m. on Saturday night.

Here are my additional tips for handling the spring forward...

- Make sure you have your room darkening shades or blackout blinds in place to shut out every last chink of daylight. With lighter mornings and evenings, our children can get confused and think it is not time to be in bed. If you need a small amount of light in your child's room go for a low watt, amber night light.

- Go outside! Exposing your children to some natural light in the daytime works wonders for their internal clocks. If you can't get outside, bright light indoors will do.
- Watch for those sleepy cues and put your child down as soon as you see the signs. These might not occur quite as you are used to with the time change so be extra vigilant.
- An earlier bedtime is actually more likely to help your child sleep in longer.
- If your child is overtired by bedtime, an emergency catnap of no more than 30 minutes and at no later than 4 p.m., could help them through and set them up for a better night's sleep.
- A day/night clock is great for a toddler who needs to know when it is time to get up or stay in bed. Visit the Products page on my website.
- Finally, don't forget to get yourself to bed early on Saturday night as well. We lose an hour in the night and you want to be well-rested to deal with a potentially tired little one as he adjusts to the change.

Fall Back – Clock change:

If your child's bedtime is normally 7 p.m., on Saturday night try to keep your child up for an extra hour and make 8 p.m. bedtime for that one night only. When the clocks change in the night, you gain an hour, so ideally your child will wake at their usual time (i.e. 7 a.m.) by the new clock time, and still have had his usual amount of sleep. Then, on Sunday night just continue with your 7 p.m. bedtime by the new clock time.

Sounds simple enough right? The difficulty might come if your child struggles to make it through to 8 p.m. on the Saturday night without becoming too overtired and grumpy and then that could lead to night waking or an unusually early start! So if this might happen for your child, you can:

- Add in a short nap in the afternoon, if he no longer naps.
- Add in an extra catnap in the afternoon for a child who is napping anyway.

OR

You can try the Split the Difference approach:

If you split the difference, you put your child to bed at 7.30 p.m. rather than stretching out to 8 p.m. He may wake a little early by the new clock time but will get back into rhythm very quickly as you will return to a 7 p.m. bedtime on Sunday night by the new clock time.

The other option you may have heard about is the gradual approach where you move the child's bedtime in 15 minute increments over the four days preceding the clock change. This works well for some people but I think it can become quite confusing and not necessarily be of much benefit to the child.

The gradual approach works like this:

Wednesday night bedtime is 7.15 p.m.

Thursday night bedtime is 7.30 p.m.

Friday night bedtime is 7.45 p.m.

Saturday night bedtime is 8 p.m. (Then the clocks go back in the middle of the night.)

Sunday night bedtime is the new 7 p.m.

Many children are not affected by a small difference in time so it is simpler and perhaps easier to make a quick adjustment by doing the immediate shift. You know your child best and you will know what will work for you but to avoid a horribly early wake-up call on Sunday morning, I do suggest you have a plan in place.

Imperfect Parenting

Being there, being present and responsive and emotionally available are the most important things you can do for your child. With so many of us hearing what other parents are doing through social media, baby groups and friends, it is easy to feel overwhelmed and confused and even wonder if you are 'getting it right'. The truth is there is no right way to do things. Parenting is unique to every parent and every family. Usually we all have the same base objectives to love and care for our children and provide them with warmth, shelter and security, to educate them, to enjoy them and to give them a happy home and family life. *How* you go about it is up to you and it may not be the same as every other parent you talk to.

Many years ago it was quite common for the men to go out to work while the women stayed at home. Maintaining the home and family duties can be quite challenging alone but in our modern society, women and mothers often juggle a lot more at once. Looking after the family home, caring for the children, maintaining a healthy marriage and holding down a career. Many women feel they need to appear like they have it all handled at all times. I am sure you have met a mother or two who just seem to have it all and with a cherry on top! Well don't let that immaculate house, those well behaved children, the blissful marriage and the nice career faze you because I assure you, things are never as 'perfect' as they seem. We are all human after all. It is often those who feel the need to always appear 'perfect' and in control, who are actually wearing a mask to hide their insecurities, self doubts, worries and fears.

So next time you feel like every other mum at the group has a baby who is sleeping through the night or all your friends who are parents seem to be finding it easy and enjoying every second – instead of wondering 'what is wrong with me?', start wondering what is their reality? What truths are they hiding? If you are genuine, authentic and vulnerable, you will find that others around you might start to be as well. Surround yourself with those who will support each other rather than compete with each other and you will feel the pressure lift off your shoulders.

Your USP (Unique Sleep Plan™):

Now that you have a good understanding of your child's sleep needs, you can transfer the information into your very own USP (Unique Sleep Plan) which will serve as a handy guide that you can turn to when you need a reminder.

Child's Name: _____ Today's Date: _____

Child's Age: _____

Identifying the causes

Do we have a bedtime routine which includes the same steps, in the same order and at the same time every evening?

How much help do we give our child to get to sleep?
(Circle any that apply)

Rocking?   Holding hand?

Feeding?   Rubbing/Patting?

Singing/Music?   Walking around?

Staying with him/her?   Holding/cuddling?

Other _____

Does my child go to bed awake and settle himself to sleep without any help at all from me?

Does my child settle himself back to sleep if he wakes up in the night, without any help, calling out or getting up?

Does my child take enough daytime sleep?
Look at The Sleep Nanny's chart on page 75 to see the average daytime sleep amounts for each age. If your child is falling beneath the average sleep amount, she is likely to be overtired.

Fill in the blanks to help you remember:

_____ is the number one cause of night _____ and _____

Knowing what an ideal schedule looks like for my child:
Look at The Sleep Nanny's chart on page 75 and complete the following:

My child requires, on average, the following amount of sleep:

Total amount of night-time sleep   _____
Total amount of daytime sleep   _____
Number of naps   _____

My child's wakeful window is approximately _____ (mins/hrs) long.

A bedtime routine is most effective when it lasts around ____ minutes.

Most children do well with a bedtime somewhere between _____ and _____ p.m.

Creating my child's sleep plan

We aim to work toward an approximate schedule as follows:

Sleep Summary

My child's day starts at   _____ a.m.
1st nap at   _____ a.m. (if applicable)
2nd nap at   _____ p.m. (if applicable)
3rd nap at   _____ p.m. (if applicable)
Bedtime routine should start at   _____ p.m.
Asleep by   _____ p.m.

Our bedtime routine will consist of these steps:

_____

_____

_____

_____

_____

Our bedtime plan:

_____

_____

_____

_____

_____

_____

If using Sleep Manners Chart, our sleep manners will be:

_____

_____

_____

_____

If using the fading technique, our chair positions will be:

Nights 1-3   _____

Nights 4-6   _____

Nights 7-9   _____

Nights 10-12   _____

Our night-time response plan:

Will you be feeding your child during the night?
    If yes, note the feeding plan and who will be implementing it.

_____

_____

_____

_____

_____

_____

Our nap plan: (We will begin nap coaching _____)

_____

_____

_____

_____

_____

_____

Our nap time routine will be between _____ and _____ minutes long and consist of:

1._____

2._____

3._____

Our backup nap plan is:

_____

_____

_____

Share nap plan with day care provider if necessary.

Implementation

The hardest part of any plan is implementing it. It can all make perfect sense on paper but actually *doing* it is a different story. To see your desired results, it is time to commit to implementing your plan with total consistency.

I'm ready to tackle this and have cleared the diary of any major outings, trips or events for a period of three weeks. Night one of our plan will be on _____

Support

Support during sleep training is incredibly valuable especially when the going gets tough. Join the Sleep Nanny's Facebook community in The Sleep Centre www.facebook.com./groups/sleepcentre to ask questions, share experiences and connect with fellow parents who are having similar experiences to you.

Beyond This Book

If you would like further information about The Sleep Nanny® and the products and services available to you, please visit us:

www.sleepnanny.co.uk

A Gift For All Readers!

The Sleep Nanny® would like to offer you a FREE guide, 'Born To Sleep' - 5 ways to get your child to sleep and what you are doing to sabotage this. Get your copy right now at:

www.sleepnanny.co.uk/borntosleep

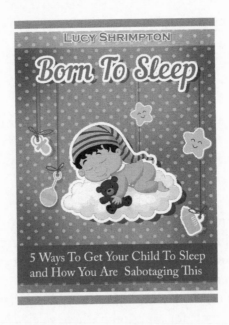

Printed in Great Britain
by Amazon.co.uk, Ltd.,
Marston Gate.